Mediterranean Diet for Beginners

Healthy weight loss in 30 days while still eating delicious food

By Christina J Evans

© Copyright 2021 by Christina J Evans - All rights reserved.

The content contained within this book may not be reproduced, duplicated, or transmitted without direct written permission from the author or the publisher.

Under no circumstances will any blame or legal responsibility be held against the publisher, or author, for any damages, reparation, or monetary loss due to the information contained within this book. Either directly or indirectly.

Legal Notice:

This book is copyright protected. This book is only for personal use. You cannot amend, distribute, sell, use, quote, or paraphrase any part, or the content within this book, without the consent of the author or publisher.

Disclaimer Notice:

Please note the information contained within this document is for educational and entertainment purposes only. All effort has been executed to present accurate, up-to-date, and reliable, complete information. No warranties of any kind are declared or implied. Readers acknowledge that the author is not engaging in the rendering of legal, financial, medical, or professional advice. The content within this book has been derived from various sources. Please consult a licensed professional before attempting any techniques outlined in this book

By reading this document, the reader agrees that under no circumstances is the author responsible for any losses, direct or indirect, which are incurred as a result of the use of the information contained within this document, including, but not limited to, — errors, omissions, or inaccuracies.

Table of Contents

Introduction 10

Chapter 1 13

Understanding the Mediterranean Diet 13

    Important Features of the Mediterranean Diet 14

    The History of the Mediterranean Diet 15

    Scientific Research on the Mediterranean Diet 16

Chapter 2 19

Mediterranean Lifestyle and Benefits 19

    Key Food Groups 19

        ➢ Vegetables 19

        ➢ Fruits 21

        ➢ Fats 21

        ➢ Lentils 22

        ➢ Wholegrains 22

        ➢ Fish 23

        ➢ Dairy 23

        ➢ Red Meat 24

    Mealtimes are Get-Together Times 25

    Exercise is the Key 25

Health Benefits of the Mediterranean Diet 26

Chapter 3 29

Planning your Mediterranean Diet 29

Planning Your Mediterranean Diet 29

Steps to Get Started with the Mediterranean Diet 32

The Mediterranean Diet Food List 35

Tips For Success on The Mediterranean Diet 45

Chapter 4 49

What to look out for in your Mediterranean Diet 49

Eating Out on The Mediterranean Diet 49

30 Days Meal Plan 53

Meal Prep Tips 65

Chapter 5 69

Sauces, Dips, and Dressings 69

Tzatziki Sauce 69

Tahini Sauce 70

Italian Red Pesto 72

Salsa Verde 73

Baba Ganoush 74

Lebanese Hummus 75

Guacamole 76

Roasted Tomato Spread (Matbucha) 78

Pickled Mango Sauce 79

Cherry Tomato Sauce 81

Roasted Red Pepper Dip (Muhammara) 82

Ranch Dressing 83

Tangy Italian Salad Dressing 84

Yogurt Tahini Dressing 85

Balsamic, Dill and Yogurt Dressing 87

Chapter 6 89

Breakfast 89

Greek-Style Frittata 89

Spinach and Goat Cheese Quiche 91

Mini Quiche with Spinach and Mushroom 92

Baked Eggs in Avocado 94

Avocado Toast with Egg 95

Zucchini with Egg 96

Shakshuka 97

Cherry and Walnut Overnight Oats 99

Blackberry and Ginger Overnight Bulgur 100

Quinoa and Chia Oatmeal Mix 101

Quinoa with Blueberry and Lemon 102

Yogurt with Blueberries and Honey ... 104

Chapter 7 ... 105

Lunch ... 105

    Tuna Patties ... 105

    Mediterranean Salmon ... 106

    Shrimp Linguine ... 107

    Vegetarian Pasta Carbonara ... 109

    Bean Burgers ... 110

    Herby Black Bean Salad with Feta Cheese ... 112

    Tomato, Basil, and Chickpea Salad ... 113

    Tabouli Salad ... 114

    Roasted Eggplants ... 115

    Mediterranean Cauliflower Pizza ... 117

    Quinoa and Avocado Salad ... 119

    Chickpea and Quinoa Bowl ... 120

Chapter 8 ... 122

Snacks ... 122

    Pineapple and Green Smoothie ... 122

    Tahini and Date Shake ... 123

    Chia and Pomegranate Smoothie ... 124

    Mediterranean Fruit Salad ... 126

Trail Mix 127

Flatbread Crackers 128

Roasted Chickpeas 130

Fish Sticks 132

Chapter 9 137

Dinner 137

Cod with Tomatoes and Olives 137

Shrimp in Garlic Sauce 140

Greek Turkey Burgers 141

Grilled Chicken Kabobs 142

Sweet and Sour Chicken 144

Hasselback Caprese Chicken 145

Lentil, Chickpea and Tomato Soup 147

Greek Red Lentil Soup 148

Greek Pasta 150

Roasted Tomato and Basil Soup 153

Chapter 10 155

Desserts 155

Olive Oil Gelato 155

Chocolate Avocado Mousse 157

Rice Pudding with Almond Milk 158

Vanilla Baked Pears 159

Strawberry Popsicles 160

Coconut, Tahini, and Cashew Bars 161

Applesauce Oat Muffins 163

Baked Apple Slices 164

Chocolate Dipped Strawberries 166

Watermelon and Mint Granita 167

Peach Soup 168

Grilled Watermelon Salad 169

Conclusion 172

My other books you will love! 174

Don't forget to grab your GIFT!!! 175

References 176

Just for You

A free gift to our readers

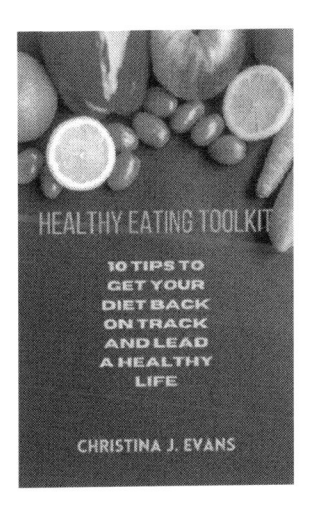

Click here

http://christinajevans.com/healthy-eating.pdf

Joining the HL Community

Looking to build your healthy eating lifestyle? If so, then check out the Healthy Living (HL) Community here:

www.facebook.com/groups/1004091000384321/

Introduction

It is a general consensus that if you eat healthily, you will live a longer and more fulfilling life, but people find it really hard to stick with diets or with eating healthy because it asks you to make an effort which is not easy if you are living a fast-paced life. The people who do try to make an effort are unable to sustain it for more than 6 months simply because there is no pleasure in eating bland and tasteless food. If you are eating healthy, but your physical and mental health is still suffering, then is it worth it? This is why the Mediterranean diet is so different from other diets. It is not just a diet; it is a way of living.

Fast food has become a go-to meal because it's quick, cheap, and you don't have to put in an effort to eat it. A study conducted on childhood obesity proved that fast food was linked to a higher BMI (Body Mass Index) score, a higher body fat percentage, and a higher chance of obesity (K.Fraser, 2012). This is true because whether you believe it or not, food has a lot of control over how we feel, and eating fast food is not pleasurable. Research has also proven that eating fast food leads to depression or an increased risk of depression (Sánchez-Villegas, 2011). Of course, when you live a fast-paced life because you are constantly working and eating unfulfilling food that does not enrich your body, this results in a lifestyle that starts weighing on you over time.

"I have been on a diet for 2 weeks, and all I have lost is 14 days." – Totie Fields

I think we all have had times when we suddenly wake up one day and want to live a healthier lifestyle. Perhaps your health is declining due to the added weight, or you aren't as fit as you used to be. In any case, you want to try and live a healthier life so you can live for longer without increasing your risk of heart disease and high blood pressure. The problem is, losing weight is by no means an easy task, but sometimes, it is a necessity, and diets can be incredibly difficult, especially if you don't know the right way to go as there are many choices especially when you still want to be able to enjoy your meals.

I first started dieting because I was extremely conscious of my body weight and was insecure about my body fat. My immunity was lower because of my unhealthy eating habits, and I was getting sick more often. I decided to research healthy eating options not only because of my body weight but also to get healthier, especially since I know how hard it is to get out of eating unhealthy food once you get into it. While it may seem like changing your diet is a simple thing, people who have actually made the change or attempted to make a change know how hard it really is, considering that your whole lifestyle now revolves around how, what, and where you eat.

To be honest, I struggled a lot when I first started to diet. I couldn't really find a suitable diet plan, and when I found one, it felt like I was torturing myself because all the recipes were either really hard to recreate or bland and tasteless. I am a foodie, and there is no doubt that I love food, so when I started to diet, my primary goal was to create healthy food that wouldn't ask me to compromise on taste. That is when I started to get into the Mediterranean diet, which I knew would be best suited for my situation. It helps you lose weight and is also incredibly healthy for you since it uses a lot of fresh vegetables, herbs, nuts, and fish. In addition, the Mediterranean diet doesn't ask you to eliminate certain ingredients that are usually considered "bad," such as red meat. Instead, the diet lowers your consumption, which makes the diet a lot more enjoyable since you aren't compromising on your favorite foods.

The Mediterranean diet originated in the countries that border the Mediterranean Sea, and it is not a diet at all; rather, it is a way of life and a culinary tradition that focuses on using fresh vegetables and fruits with fresh protein. The diet uses local and sustainable ingredients to promote a natural and healthy life. There is a heavy focus on seafood and olive oil or olives in this diet, and that is because these ingredients are locally available in the region; hence they are "fresh." The premise of the diet itself is simple – eat whole foods that are in season and fresh and avoid processed foods with additives.

The Mediterranean diet has a lot of health benefits: it lowers the risk of cardiovascular disease because it contains a lot more minerals and vitamins than typical processed foods, there is also a correlation between the Mediterranean diet and a longer lifespan since the diet contains an abundance of nutrition and antioxidants which can fight the signs of aging, and most of all, the Mediterranean diet can help you lose and manage weight especially if you pair it with physical activity and lots of exercises.

We will be exploring topics on how you can switch to a sustainable healthy lifestyle which includes Mediterranean diets. I will provide a step-by-step guide that will help you make the switch to the Mediterranean diet much easier. The Mediterranean diet used to be based on the Mediterranean diet pyramid. In recent years, the U.S. guide to healthy eating has changed, which means that now the healthy way of eating includes half a plate of fruit and veggies while the other half should have protein, grains, and dairy. The U.S. guide is updated every 5 years, and currently, the core elements that make up a healthy diet are – all kinds of vegetables, fruits, grain, protein foods, and oils. We will discuss this in greater detail in the relevant chapters. (*Dietary Guide for Americans 2020-2025,*

2020). Aside from that, you will get to learn different culinary techniques and learn how to modify the diet to fit ingredients that might be available for you locally, and of course, you will find tons of new and delicious recipes.

If you have been struggling to adhere to a healthy way of eating and want to stress less about your health, the Mediterranean diet is the solution. It is not only easy and fast to prepare, but it is also inexpensive. And, if you want to live a life free of health issues without having to sacrifice flavor, then read on!

To your healthy living,

Christina J. Evans

Female Body Fat Expert | Healthy Living Advocate

Chapter 1

Understanding the Mediterranean Diet

The Mediterranean diet has been the talk of the town for quite a long time now and obviously for all the right reasons. Due to its high magnitude of health benefits, it enjoys the status of Heart-healthy by the Mayo Clinic. According to UNESCO, the Mediterranean diet has surpassed all the other diets in terms of health benefits and sustainability. In 2010, it recognized the Mediterranean diet as the "Cultural Heritage of The Mediterranean Countries" like Spain, Greece, Italy, and Morocco.

In 2020, the Mediterranean diet was voted the best diet of 2020 nutrition professionals. With all its popularity, many people have rushed to adopt the Mediterranean diet without fully understanding how it works and their efforts ended up in failure. This is because every diet faces a misconception. Saying farewell to your regular diet and switching completely to a different diet may lead to a whole new problem. The perceived help you get, in the form of articles, cookbooks, or dietitians, doesn't properly shed light on what the Mediterranean diet might mean, and obviously, the information is overwhelming. You are not sure of the right direction to follow. So here comes the very basic but burning question – WHAT EXACTLY IS THE MEDITERRANEAN DIET?!

Let's start with the word 'diet.' The word diet immediately makes you think of cutting down on food, counting calories and starving your stomach. That is the association we have been conditioned to because all the famous diets such as the Ketogenic diet and Atkins diet operate on low-carbs and high protein. These diets were created with the purpose of helping people lose weight. The latter diet helped people in their weight loss journey, but the weight was regained as soon as people switched to their normal eating habits. This is why the world needed a sustainable diet that could become a part of their lifestyle, and that's where the Mediterranean diet comes in.

The Mediterranean diet is not a diet at all but a lifestyle of the people living in Mediterranean countries. It is a culinary heritage of Mediterranean people that emphasizes the consumption of fresh fruits and seasonal vegetables. The Mediterranean diet is not about restricting food and does not focus on tracking calories. Instead, this lifestyle change aims to help you successfully eliminate unhealthy foods from your life while adding in more whole ones. It is also important to consider how these dietary changes affect habits and relationships with friends and family members. The Mediterranean diet emphasizes eating fresh seasonal foods grown locally. Whole grains, healthy fats, legumes, beans, fish, and dairy, make up a majority of the rest of the diet.

Some Mediterranean regions incorporate a great deal more legumes and lentils, while others may enjoy more whole grains options. The similarity, however, is that all these regions enjoy plenty of plant-based foods and limit processed foods as well as added sugars and refined foods from their diets. Each region consumes nearly 2 to 3 times as many fruits and vegetables compared to those on the western diet. They also eat healthy fats like olive oil, nuts, and seeds regularly.

Important Features of the Mediterranean Diet

- A majority of the Mediterranean diet consists of fresh produce like organic fruits and vegetables.
- Whole grains like barley, millet, and whole-wheat add a unique flavor to your meal with their nutty texture. These nutritious grains are enjoyed as side dishes but could be incorporated into main courses too.
- Beans, lentils, and legumes make up a significant source of protein in the Mediterranean diet. These foods tend to make up for the limited consumption of red meats.
- Chicken, turkey, duck, and fish are good lean meat options that you can load up on your plate a few times per week. Lean meats (white meat) have lower calories and less saturated fats than red meat options. And that's why lean meats make the Mediterranean diet apt for weight reduction.
- Seafood such as scallops, shrimps, prawns, lobster e.t.c are incorporated into weekly meals at least twice a week.
- Another option for protein is red meat, but it should be the last option. This is because red meats contain saturated fat and cholesterol, which contribute to increased blood cholesterol levels and may cause heart ailments. So, have red meats only once a month and make sure they are grass-fed. A nice and

delicious way to incorporate red meat in the Mediterranean diet is baking the meat with herbs and grill, not deep-frying.
- Drinking red wine in moderation is considered healthy on this diet and may help to lower the risk of heart disease. A glass or two per day has been shown to benefit your health overall.

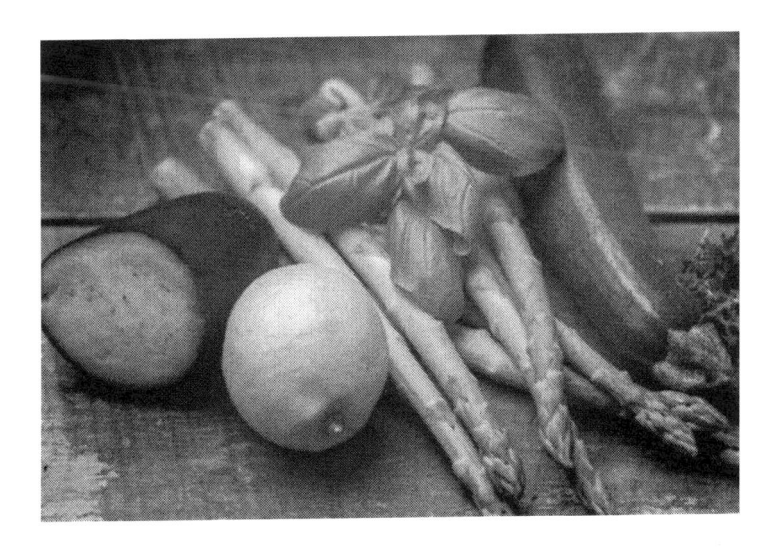

The History of the Mediterranean Diet

Many cultures have lived around the Mediterranean Sea, and their diet is important. One of their most important achievements has been the Mediterranean diet. It is hard to pinpoint where the Mediterranean originated since the eating habits that fall under this go far back into the Middle Ages.

People began farming in the areas surrounding the Mediterranean Sea, including countries like Lebanon, Israel, Palestine, Syria, and Jordan. They grew cereals and legumes. Later on, people from other countries came to live there, like Greeks and Romans. These people began to cultivate three basic food groups of the Mediterranean diet, such as olive trees for olive oil, wheat for bread, and grapevines, for the production of grapes and its main fermentation product, wine. The richer cast of Ancient Rome loved fresh fish and seafood with a special focus on oysters - either raw or fried in olive oil, while the middle or lower-middle class of Rome, including slaves, consumed foods that consisted of bread served with olive oil and olives, rarely eating any meat. (Altomare, 2013).

In the 8th Century, after Christ, Moors occupied Spain, they introduced new foods like rice and lemons to the area. These new foods gradually spread to the whole Mediterranean region. The occupation of the Moors ended in 1492, which is also when

Christopher Columbus came back from America with tomatoes and peppers. Since the 1960s, people have been interested in the eating habits of Mediterranean countries.

Scientific Research on the Mediterranean Diet

The first time people started investigating the Mediterranean diet was back in 1948 when a study was carried out on the constituents of the diet to prove its positive and negative impacts on overall health. This attempt was later rectified in 1952 by Ancel Keys, who sought to explore seven countries and their diet. The seven countries include the USA, Japan, Italy, Greece, Finland, the Netherlands, and Yugoslavia. The study spanned over three decades and evaluated data of 12,000 men aged 40 to 59. The results linked dietary intake with serum cholesterol levels and cardiovascular diseases, while low rates of cardiovascular diseases were linked to participants who had lower consumption of saturated fats. Another research conducted by the European Atomic Energy Commission, which took place from 1963 to 1965, sought to research the food consumption in 11 regions across six countries, nine regions in Northern Europe and two regions in Southern Europe. The only difference in their dietary patterns was in total fat intake where olive oil was its main source in the southern regions while butter was preferred in the northern regions. Margarine wasn't part of their diet and that's why the research found that the people in Northern and Southern Europe were also at less risk of suffering from chronic diseases. That is why, following this study, the potential effect of the Mediterranean diet, on reducing chronic diseases, was widely accepted. (Sahyoun, 2016)

After Ancel Keys, many people have conducted intensive research on the Mediterranean diet and its health benefits, including an increased lifespan, healthy weight, and improved brain function, fewer symptoms of rheumatoid arthritis, and eye health, lower risk of certain types of cancers, lower risk of heart disease, Alzheimer's, diabetes, and finally, lower blood pressure and LDL cholesterol levels. In fact, the Lyon Diet Trial proved that after three years of the continuous Mediterranean diet, the subjects showed a 50 percent lower risk of death and 50 to 70 percent reduced risk of myocardial infarction. Another research that gained worldwide attention was done by researchers in Spain who found that the Mediterranean diets, which included nuts, reduced the risk of cardiovascular diseases by 30 percent and decreased the risk of stroke by 49 percent. (Altomare, 2013)

From 2010 and onwards, many experts and doctors have recommended the Mediterranean diet for patients trying to lose weight or improve their overall wellbeing. Since then, it has been hailed as one of the best diets around. The amazing thing about the Mediterranean diet is that it doesn't credit one food or vegetable for the decreased health problems and weight loss but rather the whole plant-based diet with a special focus on local, regional, and locally available rich foods as a whole create a rich environment within the body and is responsible for all these reduced health problems. (Altomare, 2013)

As I have stated previously, the Mediterranean diet has been the focus of many research studies, and we already know about the multitude of health benefits it has. Aside from these, the Mediterranean diet is also used for weight loss. One research called "Mediterranean Diet and Weight Loss: Meta-Analysis of Randomized Controlled Trials" observed 1848 people on a Mediterranean diet and 1588 people on a controlled diet. The people who were following the Mediterranean diet showed a significant difference in weight and body mass index. The difference was observed mainly through energy restriction and increased physical activity. In no part of the study did any participant report gaining any weight, so through this study, we can conclude that the Mediterranean diet will be useful in losing weight, especially if it is accompanied by physical activity such as exercise and is longer than 6 months or is at least 6 months in duration. (Esposito, 2011)

Another research titled Systematic Review of the Mediterranean Diet for Long-Term Weight Loss supported the results of our previous research. It looked at the long-term benefits of the Mediterranean diet in obese and overweight participants. In the trials, the Mediterranean diet was compared to a low-fat diet, a low-carbohydrate diet, and the American diabetes association diet. The people in the Mediterranean diet group showed greater weight loss than the low-fat diet at 12 months. The Mediterranean diet also improved the cardiovascular risk factor levels, including blood pressure and lipid levels. (G. Mancini, 2016)

Over the last few decades, we have accumulated enough evidence that supports the fact that dietary habits have a large impact on the occurrence of diseases. The major scientific associations such as WHO, world health organization emphasize the role of diet in preventing non-communicable diseases. Many studies noticed that foods such as fruits and vegetables, fibers and whole grains with fish, and moderate alcohol consumption reduced the risk of major degenerative diseases and the food groups that are usually associated with that fall under the Mediterranean diet. Similarly, the Mediterranean diet has been associated with a more favorable health outcome and a better quality of life. (Sofi, 2015)

The Mediterranean diet is created by a centuries-old tradition that is associated with excellent health and provides a sense of pleasure and wellbeing. It, in a sense, forms a vital part of the world's collective cultural heritage. The Mediterranean diet has several characteristics: an abundance of plant foods, olive oil as the principal fat, dairy products mostly yogurt and cheese, red meat, poultry, fish, and eggs in moderate amounts, moderate wine, and physical activity. For Mediterranean people, the diet is a way of living that needs to be revitalized in modern times, and people who want to follow such a diet are intrigued and attracted because of the strong palatability and the health benefits that are associated with the diet. The meals can be either recreated on their own or take into account different cultures and the feasibility of local ingredients. (Willet, 1995)

I want to believe that by now, you have successfully gathered "WHAT ACTUALLY A MEDITERRANEAN DIET IS." In the next chapter, you will find all the necessary information to satisfy your every possible "WHY THE MEDITERRANEAN DIET" question. I am sure that the research would be more than enough for you to easily incorporate the elements of the Mediterranean lifestyle diet into your life. You can even tailor the Mediterranean diet according to your native cuisine, and like me, you can also enjoy the best of both worlds!!!

Chapter 2

Mediterranean Lifestyle and Benefits

The major part of the Mediterranean lifestyle emphasizes the consumption of plant-based foods into your diet. The main components of the Mediterranean lifestyle include generous eating of fresh vegetables, fruits, legumes, whole grains, fish, and mindful consumption of dairy products, white and red meat. With these food options, the Mediterranean diet lifestyle ensures that your body gets all the required nutrients to keep it healthy and wealthy while boosting your immune system. Moreover, once the body's nutrient requirements have been achieved, you will naturally feel satiated, and therefore, will not feel the need to retreat to processed foods. This chapter will discuss the benefits of the Mediterranean lifestyle but before we go into that, it is important that you know the key food groups that make up the Mediterranean diet and make it apt to lead a healthy lifestyle.

Key Food Groups

- Vegetables

Fresh vegetables constitute a major part of the Mediterranean diet. To retain most of the nutrients and vitamins, vegetables are eaten uncooked or slightly cooked. Bitter green vegetables like spinach, kale, or broccoli are some of the nutritious veggies that are included in this diet. These vegetables are highly rich in Vitamin A, K, and C. Besides, vegetables are also loaded with high amounts of omega-3 fatty acids. These acids are proven to be extremely beneficial for improving digestion and mitigating the chances of constipation. The amazing thing about vegetables is the fact that they are always in the season. Thus, you are never going to run out of choices.

Most of the Mediterranean meals consist of the vegetables cooked in one or the other way, and on very rare occasions, meat is included; otherwise, it is all green on the plate. Perpetually on dinners, the vegetables are served as either grilled, sauteed, or roasted.

Sometimes, salads are eaten too, along with them served as side dishes. On this diet, picking vegetables is considered a serious matter. Habitants of Mediterranean regions grow their vegetable farms and then handpick the fresh and best ones. If you do not have a farm, then it is nothing to worry about. You can always go to the local vegetable shops as they receive fresh stock almost every day directly from the farms. The reason behind choosing organic and freshly grown vegetables is that they are highly rich in nutrients. Thus, it is evident that the Mediterranean diet is all about eating locally grown fresh vegetables. You might also go overboard and buy all the organic produce but never forget that you can always freeze the vegetables in plastic bags and use them when needed.

It is important to know that canned vegetables can never be the substitute for organically grown ones. Although they have all the characteristics to tempt you, like cheap prices and quick-cooking but very low in nutrients and contain extra salt/sugar added as preservatives. So, if you wholeheartedly want to adopt the Mediterranean lifestyle, you will have to part ways with canned foods. Still, you can always use canned veggies packed in water with little to no salt/sugar. In addition to the above facts, it is recommended that you bring diversity. Simply put, do not limit yourself to some specific vegetables; instead, eat whatever seasonal vegetables are available to you.

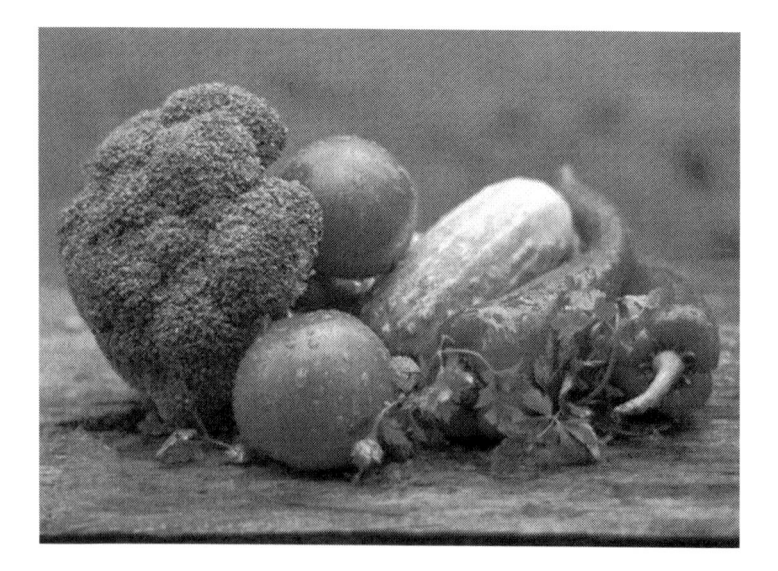

➤ Fruits

Regular fruit intake on the Mediterranean diet is a must. On this diet, fruits work as the replacement for desserts. They provide enough sugar rush that keeps you away from satisfying your sweet tooth with regular sugar-laden treats. Fruits are usually eaten for breakfast and sometimes as snacks, too, if hunger persists. Fruits can also be preserved or frozen to later use in ice cream and smoothies.

The Mediterranean diet also encourages the consumption of citrus fruits. Lemon juice is used as the most significant part of Mediterranean food. Its juice can be squished into your curry to give it a citric taste. There are no hard and fast rules to eat fruits that are purely grown in the Mediterranean region; the gist of the Mediterranean diet is to eat seasonal and fresh fruits that you can find locally in your region.

➤ Fats

The Mediterranean diet is primarily about using mono-saturated fats like olive oil. In simple terms, healthy fats. However, you should know that not all fats are similar and healthy. Some types of fats are very rich in bad cholesterol that can potentially destroy your heart health. While other types of fats are unsaturated and do not stick to your muscles, thereby reducing the chances of weight gain. Olive oil is one such example, which is the backbone of Mediterranean food, and that's why the majority of the Mediterranean recipes are cooked in olive oil. The reason is that olive oil helps with digestion and carries out maximum nutrient absorption, and helps you feel satiated.

The taste of olive oil varies from country to country. For example, olive oil in Mediterranean countries is flavorful and rich in taste. Whereas olive oil produced in America is slightly tasteless. But this must not excuse you from cooking your food in olive oil because of taste or no taste; it is healthy for you in many ways.

Besides, olive oil, another rich source of healthy fats on the Mediterranean diet, is driven from coconut, almonds, walnuts, and chia seeds. These nuts are rich in magnesium, vitamin E, and protein. Consuming enough of these nuts will ensure that you never end up in a hospital bed due to heart malfunction-related causes or diabetes.

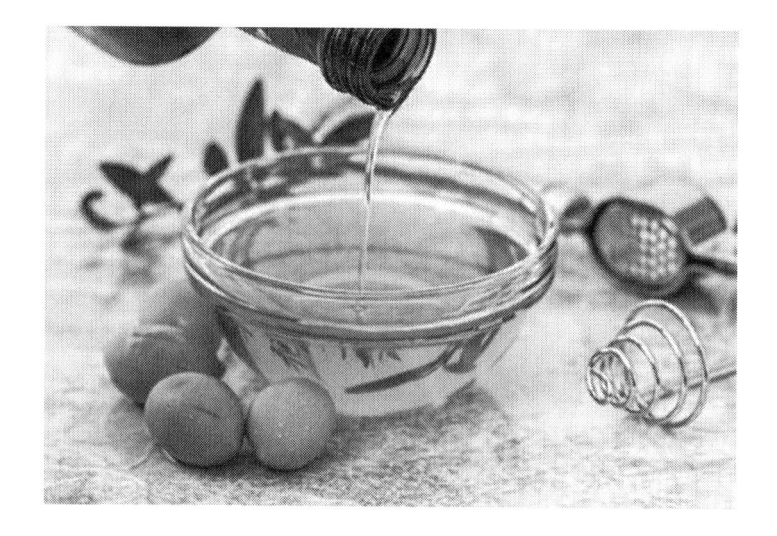

➤ Lentils

Legumes are the replacement for meat on the Mediterranean diet because they are a rich source of protein. It is seen that Mediterranean regions consume more lentils as compared to America; this is because many Mediterranean habitants observe fasts for quite a bit of time in the year, and during those days, they abstain from eating meat. This precisely explains the large consumption of lentils by Mediterranean people. Chickpeas, beans, and white beans are largely eaten on the Mediterranean diet, and these can easily be found in America. Contrary to people's belief, lentils are easy and quick to cook, given that you soak them for a while before cooking.

➤ Wholegrains

The fundamental components of the Mediterranean diet are whole grains. Whole grains include foods like bread, pasta, and rice. It is a cooking ritual in Mediterranean regions to always have a basket of bread placed during breakfast, lunch, and dinner for everyone to share from when they sit together at mealtimes. The bread usually consumed is made of sourdough, unlike white bread that is produced with the help of yeast. Furthermore, barley and wheat are the most commonly used whole grains on the Mediterranean diet. The whole grains are served as side dishes cooked in vegetables and beans.

➢ Fish

As vegetables and fruits account for the major part of the Mediterranean diet, people often attribute this diet with no traces of seafood. But that is not true because the Mediterranean diet does allow the consumption of kinds of seafood like sardines, anchovies, but their servings are kept small and eaten only once or twice a week. Moreover, since fish has healthy oils, it has been given a separate category from red meats. Octopus and mussels are considered to be the delights of Mediterranean dinners. Their scrumptious taste makes the Mediterranean diet all more worth it.

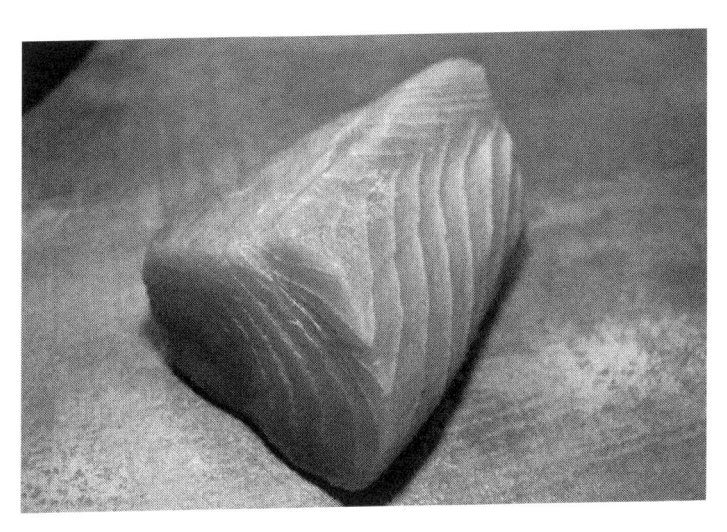

➢ Dairy

On a Mediterranean diet, consumption of dairy products is limited. Since milk and cheese tend to be high in cholesterol, their usage has been restricted to once or twice a week. By now, we know that the Mediterranean diet is all about keeping one healthy and fit, so how can it possibly allow the consumption of such fats that can potentially form fat clots in heart arteries causing a heart attack or leading to obesity. So instead, preference is given low-fat dairy items or made from plants such as almond and coconut milk, coconut yogurt, etc.

➢ Red Meat

Red meat is only eaten on special occasions when on the Mediterranean diet. It is served as a side dish instead of the main course. The servings are kept small. Its replacement includes fish, poultry, and beans. The meat of grass-fed animals can also be a viable replacement for red meat primarily because the earlier animals are healthier and eat clean. The best recommendation by the dietician is that when you want to choose meat, choose one that is 90 percent lean with 10 percent fat.

You will get more details about making your plate for the Mediterranean diet as per serving in the section "The Mediterranean Diet Food List" of chapter 3.

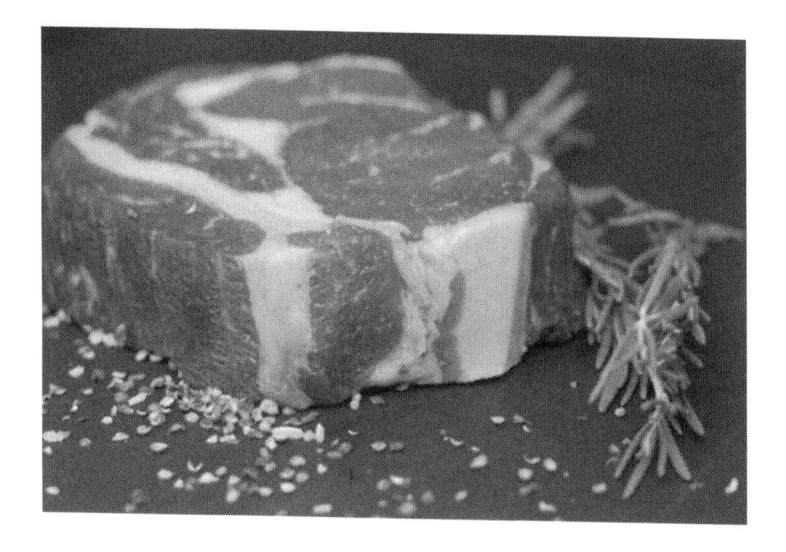

Mealtimes are Get-Together Times

Mediterranean meals are seen as a way to relax and reconnect. They transform mealtimes into an experience, encouraging family members to gather at the table for conversation instead of staying on their phones or watching T.V. in another room. In the western world, many are used to rushing through meals as fast as possible. We often approach this experience with an obligation rather than a time for reflection and connection. It is common in American homes for family members to be glued to their phones scrolling social media during dinner times. This lack of engagement leads to increased stress levels, leading one to depression or other mental health issues over long periods. An alternative solution would be putting down your devices at mealtime instead and focusing on those around you, enjoying them more fully - it will reduce stress and increase moods overall. Social eating or the act of sharing a meal with another person can reduce stress and the risk of overeating. Eating together as a family is also an opportunity to connect and support your children while also teaching them how to eat healthily.

Even though cooking is usually a solitary event, it has also been known to be social. When multiple people get together in the kitchen, they can connect and share their days' events. It is not uncommon for those invited over dinner to come early so that everyone can help cook and stay connected throughout the night.

Exercise is the Key

The Mediterranean region is an area where physical activity plays a major role in the health of its citizens. Many people there choose to walk rather than drive or take public transit all around their cities and towns. And this leads them closer with neighbors and friends. Not only that, but these regular walks play a large part in exceptional wellbeing for those who live here. Most individuals who follow the Mediterranean diet also get two hours of cardio or aerobic exercise per week. It can be split up throughout the week and done in 10-minute intervals by engaging in daily chores such as mowing your lawn, cleaning the house, vacuuming carpets, etc. You can also divide it by exercising at least two hours per week by running around with your kids for fun or even dancing.

Some exercises to consider:

- Jogging
- Swimming
- Yoga
- Running
- Walking
- Strength training
- Resistance training
- Cycling

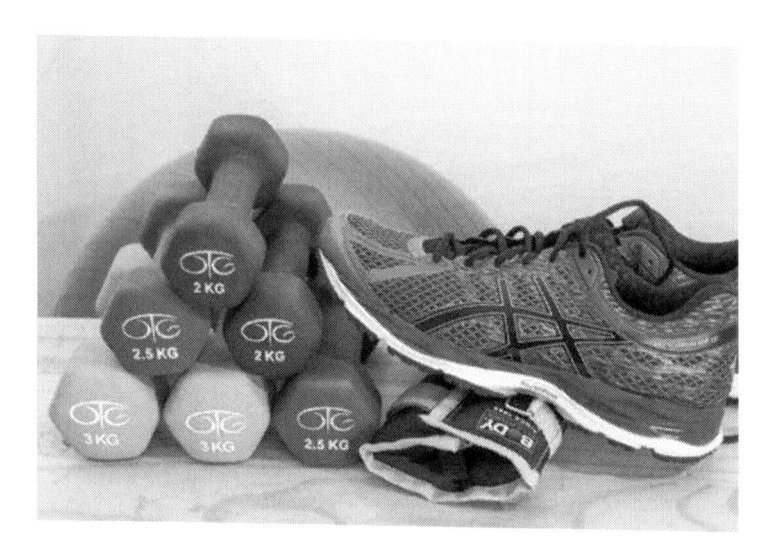

Health Benefits of the Mediterranean Diet

Let's talk about the impact of the Mediterranean lifestyle on our health. As you are aware now, the Mediterranean diet focuses on eating a variety of fruits, vegetables, nuts, healthy fats, and proteins. This healthy lifestyle has been proven to increase life expectancy by up to 10 years! Along with the benefits for your health, adopting this diet can also provide increased mental clarity because it is high in Omega-3s, which support brain function. So, if you are looking for improved mood or decreased anxiety levels, then look no further than changing how you eat. Seriously, what could be better?

The significant health benefits of the Mediterranean diet can be found below:

➤ *Strengthens Heart Health*

A large clinical trial in Spain of 7,000 people with pre-diabetes or high risk for cardiovascular disease showed that those who ate a calorie-unrestricted Mediterranean diet rich in olive oil and nuts had at least a 30 percent lower chance of heart attack. So undoubtedly, the Mediterranean diet is a wholesome, healthy way to reduce the risk of cardiovascular disease.

➤ *Minimize Women's Risk for Stroke*

A September 2018 study published in the Stroke Journal found that following a Mediterranean diet could lower the risk of stroke, especially for women at high risk. Researchers examined data on 23,232 men and women ages 40 to 77 from the United Kingdom, with most being white. The results showed a significant reduction in strokes only for female participants, not so much among males. Females experienced an average 20 percent decrease when they followed this specific diet regimen closely.

➤ *Good For Cognitive and Prevention of Brain Damage*

To provide the brain with all of its nutritional needs, people must have a rich blood supply. However, those who are experiencing vascular issues can experience significant cognitive decline as well. A July 2016 review published in the journal Frontiers in Nutrition examined studies that looked at cognitive function and concluded: *"there is encouraging evidence that a higher adherence to the Mediterranean diet improves cognition, slows cognitive decline or reduces conversion from Alzheimer's disease."*

➤ *Keeps Cancer at Bay*

The Mediterranean diet plan is considered very effective in mitigating the chances of developing certain types of cancers, such as breast cancer. New research has shown that the Mediterranean diet can help reduce your risk of breast cancer and colorectal cancers and prevent death from these types of cancer.

The Mediterranean diet is linked to lower rates of depression, according to a study published in September 2018. Analysis from four longitudinal studies revealed that the reduction was 33 percent.

> Weight Loss on the Mediterranean Diet

The Mediterranean diet, by far, provides an authentic and sure way to shed extra pounds naturally and easily. Unlike other diets like keto diets that follow the principle of low carbohydrates and more protein, the Mediterranean diet strikes a balance between all the basic nutrients required by the human body.

It does not deprive you of food like other diets; instead, it provides you with healthy food rich in antioxidants that stimulate fast metabolism, thereby quick digestion and no fat storage. In addition to that, the Mediterranean diet is clean eating where you are cutting off the sources of bad cholesterol that leads to obesity. Also, it removes fast foods from your life which are the big cause of obesity in people. The latter ensures lower calorie intake and quick satiation. Since the Mediterranean diet is rich in healthful foods and provides a high quantity of fiber and good fats, both of these lead to weight loss.

With all the information for understanding the prominent features of the Mediterranean lifestyle along with food groups and potential health advantages, it's time to dive a little deeper to comprehend your adaptation to it. The efforts you need to make for **TRANSITIONING TO THE MEDITERRANEAN DIET** are convenient and a lot easier than you can imagine!

Chapter 3

Planning your Mediterranean Diet

Like I discussed with you at the beginning of chapter 1, many people dive right into this new way of eating without planning or understanding the ins and outs of what they should be doing to achieve their goals. That is precisely what this chapter is about – planning your Mediterranean diet plate, convenient steps to get started with the diet, a detailed food list, and tricks for ensuring your success in adapting to the Mediterranean diet.

So, the transition to the diet can get a lot easier, and for this, it is necessary to gather all the information about the ingredients and their cooking techniques to make this transition easy and smooth. In addition, you should know what foods to eat, what foods to avoid and what foods to not eat at all. Even though there are no supplements or special foods to purchase, some key ingredients are a must-have on this diet, which you will be required to buy and stock up on. Moreover, you will also have to locate organic farms that could supply fresh stock of seasonal fruits and vegetables.

Transitioning to the Mediterranean diet is mostly about making yourself ready for a new way of eating. It also means adapting to the Mediterranean lifestyle and changing your relationship with food. For this journey to be merry, you will have to unlearn everything about your unhealthy eating habits and change how you look at food. It suffices to say that transitioning to the Mediterranean diet demands a change of mindset and modifying your life so that the Mediterranean diet becomes your natural eating pattern. You can take as much time as you want to prepare yourself beforehand.

Planning Your Mediterranean Diet

Unlike other fancy diets, you do not have to run stores to stores to get the right ingredients to prepare a Mediterranean dish. Ingredients of the Mediterranean diet are available almost everywhere. You are also not required to buy advanced electrical appliances to cook your food into. The only thing you have to do is find the right ingredients and get started. You need to take care of just a few things, and you will be successful on this diet. The following are some of the ways you can start mentally preparing yourself for transitioning to the Mediterranean diet.

➢ *Make Healthy Eating Effortless*

Before completely diving into the Mediterranean eating patterns, it is advisable to cut off all ties with processed, unhealthy foods. This will serve as a warm-up for you. If this goes smoothly, then you will not have much problem adjusting to the said diet. Start by completely boycotting fast foods. Then slowly start cutting on other processed food like chips, canned and frozen foods.

You can also snub on processed drinks like sodas, juices, and coffee and replace them with milk, butter, sugar. As far as frozen meat is concerned, you can replace it with a limited portion of red meat.

It may seem overwhelming to abruptly cut down these foods because your body has been using them as a source of energy for a long time. This is why it needs to be done slowly and gradually. After some time of following this regime, you will notice positive changes in your body.

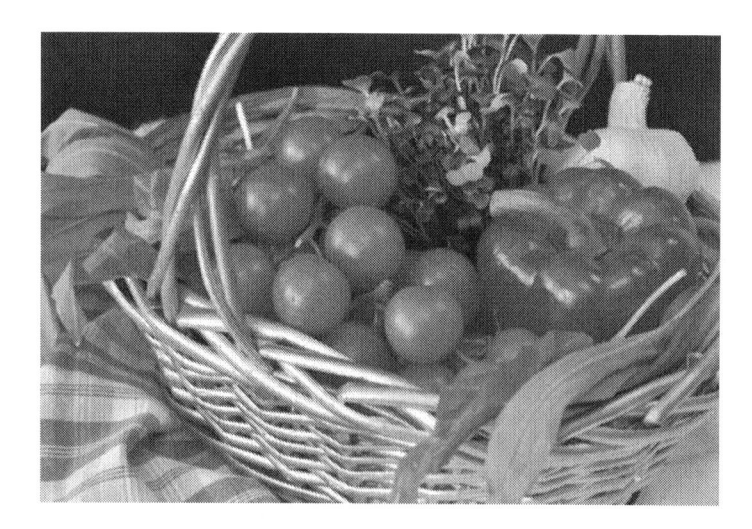

➤ *Think About the Scrumptious Mediterranean Food*

Think of Mediterranean food as like going on a vacation. When you plan for a trip, you do your homework beforehand, for example, searching for hotels, places to visit, and things to try. It builds a certain excitement and gives you a reason to look forward to. Just like that, consider practicing the Mediterranean diet as an adventure and a quest for attaining maximum health benefits. Therefore, you should educate yourself about everything related to the Mediterranean diet, for example, foods and drinks to have and avoid. Plus, cooking Mediterranean dishes will take this adventure to another level; see chapter 5 and onwards to try your cooking skills. In this manner, you will train yourself enough to ensure a successful and smooth transition.

➤ *Shop For the Ingredients*

The best part about the Mediterranean diet is that the ingredients used in it are readily available everywhere, be it supermarkets, organic farms, or even your backyard garden. Chapter 2 discussed the importance of picking your own produce, and for this, you need to make this activity a joyful quest.

All you need to do is put your coat on and be on your way to get fresh vegetables and fruits. Of course, you will have to check out the freshness and get a quote for prices too. In this manner, you will be better equipped to shop for your required ingredients. Still, the primary goal is to locate as many sources of fresh fruits, vegetables, and meat regardless of the time taken in the process. The most recommended way to source your food on the Mediterranean diet is to source it from organic farms. These farms produce fresh and healthy seasonal food. This food is not only rich in nutrition, but it tastes good as well. Also, try to befriend the vendors, so you can remain updated about the upcoming stock. You can also talk to farmers and inquire about the timings of harvests of different vegetables used on the Mediterranean diet. Befriending farmers, talking to them, and taking an interest in what they do is an amazing way to encourage healthy social interaction. The latter is part of Mediterranean culture. Besides friendship, you can get amazing discounts and updated information on the upcoming harvests too. And as you get used to shopping, the experience will be just like a trip to the park.

You can also retreat to supermarkets and grocery stores if you cannot access local farms. As long as you abide by the basic notions of the Mediterranean diet, you are on the right track. While shopping for Mediterranean ingredients, try to stay in the vicinity of the market. It implies that you should try to buy all of your ingredients from the fresh produce section, including seafood, dairy, and meat. Fill your cart with as many organic fruits and vegetables as you can because you can never have enough healthy food. These vegetables are going to be a rich source of antioxidants for you. Moreover, try to opt for in-season fruits rather than out-season. The reason is that out-season fruits usually have lost their nutritional value.

Befriend the sea monger at the seafood shop. Do this for two reasons. Firstly, you get to fill your cart with fresh fish; and secondly, he will be able to help you pick the fresh fish and even, could share scrumptious Mediterranean cooking recipes with you—all the good reasons to be friends with them. Try to choose cold water fishes as they are rich in omega-3. For example, you can go for sardines, salmon, mackerel, and cod.

In addition to that, avoid shopping for food from center aisles in the supermarkets, as these sell processed and artificial preserved canned foods, which is a big no on the Mediterranean diet. What you can only get from these aisles are oils and whole grains like pasta, bread, and walnuts. Just to be sure, keep your grocery list in hand so you don't get tempted by forbidden foods on this diet.

Steps to Get Started with the Mediterranean Diet

The primary proposition of the Mediterranean diet is to replicate the eating pattern of the Mediterranean regions. The U.S. Department of Agriculture's (USDA) My plate provides a comprehensive guideline in the "Dietary Guidelines for Americans 2020-2025" about eating healthy foods on the Mediterranean diet. You can go through the details according to your age group; however, if you still feel confused about food choices, then remember one simple rule and apply it to every meal. Make half your plate fruits and vegetables, one-quarter of your plate whole grains, one-quarter of your plate healthy protein, some dairy, and lots of water.

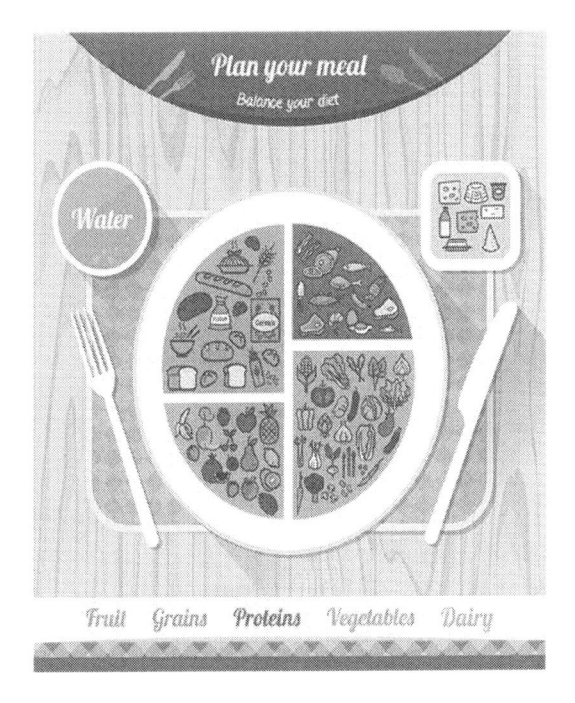

The Mediterranean lifestyle is an easy way to get back on track with your healthy eating habits. It has been found that people who live in this region have lower obesity, heart disease, and diabetes rates than the average person. Therefore, the Mediterranean diet is a great choice for anyone looking to get healthier, lower cholesterol levels, and lose weight. Now that you have been introduced to the wonders of a Mediterranean diet, it is time to show you how easy and delicious transitioning into this lifestyle can be. I will walk you through a five-step guide for making the switch from your old ways with healthy eating habits so come along on an exciting journey toward better health.

I have mentioned five steps for your ease in transitioning to the Mediterranean diet.

Step 1: When You Cook, Use Olive Oil

You must replace other fats with olive oil if you want the benefits of the Mediterranean diet. Olive oil is central to this type of diet, and many people think it has good fats. But, if you do not replace other types of fat with olive oil, then you will not get those benefits.

Step 2: Eat Vegetables as the Main Dish

One of the main features that set the Mediterranean Diet apart from most other diets is its high consumption of vegetables. Greeks consume almost a pound per day, and this can be seen in their cooking techniques, such as sautéed green beans with olive oil or tomato sauce.

Step 3: Learn to Cook Some Simple Mediterranean Meals

The Mediterranean diet is a refreshing change from the Western standard. It consists of real food that can make your life happier and healthier, like omelets with fresh vegetables or grilled fish topped with tomatoes. You might not have to cook from scratch every day, but learning 2-3 basic dishes will help you in the long run.

Step 4: Try Going Vegan for One Day A Week

It may have been that the Greeks' diet was so healthy because they abstained from animal products for roughly half of their year. This would make sense as not only a religious practice but also potentially an important factor in why this population had much better health than others at the time due to less consumption of animal-based foods and more plant-based foods.

Step 5: Do Not Add Meat to Everything

Many people see vegetables on the recommendation list, but what does meat add to a diet? Studies show that reducing your intake of red and white meats will have better health benefits. Try these guidelines: one serving of lean beef once per week and three servings of chicken weekly, one every two days, with fish as an alternative for those who do not like white or red meat.

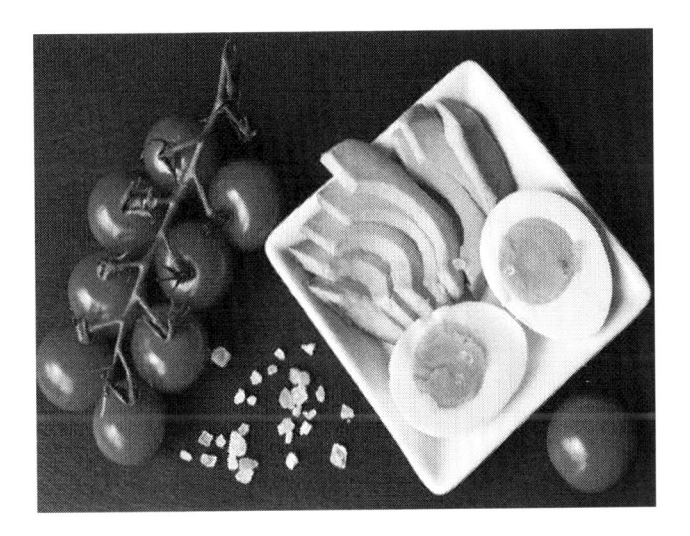

The Mediterranean Diet Food List

The Mediterranean diet is often considered a way to promote good health and longevity. The beauty of this dietary regimen lies in its never-ending food options, which, combined with the diversity of all regions, makes it rich. We need to take care of some basics when following or creating any type of Mediterranean style eating habits, such as what foods you should eat, which items to avoid, which beverages to drink, etc.

Vegetables

What to Eat liberally:

- All vegetables that are non-starchy such as dark greens, artichokes, eggplant, bell peppers, zucchini, etc.
- Brightly colored veggies such as kale, spinach, tomatoes, eggplant, squash, and okra.
- Moderately starchy vegetables such as root vegetables like carrots, beets, and sweet potatoes.
- Frozen or canned vegetables with no added sugar or salt.

What to Eat Rarely or Never:

- Vegetables that are very starchy such as white potatoes and corn.

Instructions for Servings:

At least 5 or more servings of fresh vegetables per day, such as

- make 2 servings of salad
- 1 medium vegetable
- ½ cup of canned vegetables
- 1 cup of leafy greens

Fruits

What to Eat liberally:

- All fruits that are high in fiber and low in sugar are allowed, such as berries, cherries, apricots, peaches, dates, oranges, pears, figs, melons, peaches, etc.
- Frozen or canned fruits with no added sugar or salt.
- Dried fruits with no added sugar.

What to Eat Rarely or Never:

- There is no fruit that is off-limit on the Mediterranean diet as long as it is fresh.

Instructions for Servings:

At least 3 or more servings of fresh fruit per day, such as

- have 1 medium fruit
- ½ cup of canned fruit
- ¼ cup dried fruit

Nuts and Seeds

What to Eat liberally:

Eat nuts and seeds but in moderation

What to Eat Occasionally:

- Almonds, pistachios, and cashews
- Walnuts and Hazelnut
- All unsweetened nuts

What to Eat Rarely or Never:

- Sugar-coated nuts
- Sweetened nut butter
- Sweetened trail mixes

Instructions for Servings:

- 1 serving of ¼ cup unsalted seeds or nuts per week

Whole Grains

What to Eat liberally:

- All grains that have whole or whole-grain in their name, including whole-grain wheat, whole-grain rice, etc.
- Products with whole grains as their first grain ingredients, such as whole-grain bread and whole-grain cereal
- Other grains and products include couscous, oats, barley, quinoa, bulgur, brown rice, wild rice, spelt, millet, farro, and buckwheat.

What to Eat Occasionally:

- Couscous
- Whole-wheat pasta
- Whole-grain crackers
- Polenta
- All-bran cereals

What to Eat Rarely or Never:

- Pancake mix
- Frozen waffles
- Sugar-sweetened cereals
- Crackers
- High fat snack foods like French fries, chips, buttered popcorn, cheese puffs, etc.

Instructions for Servings:

5 servings per day such as

- have ½ cup cooked grains in the form of rice or pasta
- 1 slice of wholegrain bread
- 30 grams of crackers or cold cereal
- ¾ cup hot cereal
- ½ of whole-grain roti, tortilla, or pita bread

Lentils, Beans, and Peas

What to Eat liberally:

- Red beans, kidney beans, and other beans, all lentils and pulses

Instructions for Servings:

At least 3 or more servings per week

- Make ¾ cup of cooked lentils, beans, and peas

Poultry and Red Meat

What to Eat liberally:

- Chicken, turkey, duck, game hens, eggs, and egg whites
- Plant-based alternatives of poultry such as tofu, tempeh, and seitan

What to Eat Occasionally:

- Red meat, grass-fed: beef, pork, lamb, or goat (baked, grilled)
- Bacon, grass-fed
- Processed meat products such as chicken nuggets (baked)

What to Eat Rarely or Never:

- Processed meat like ham, bacon, sausages, deli meats
- Meat cuts that are high in salt and saturated fats

Instructions for Servings:

- 2 to 5 servings of poultry per week
- 3 to 5 servings of red meat per month
- Prefer poultry to red meat

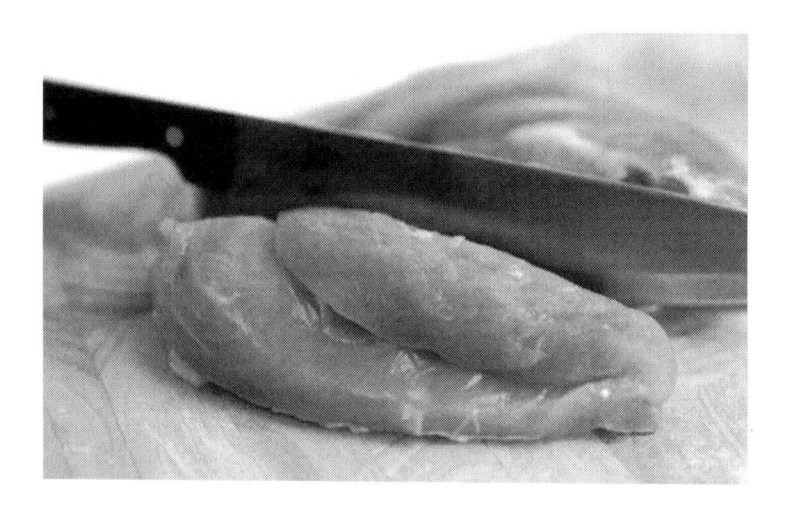

Fish and Seafood

What to Eat liberally:

- Fish that are high in omega-3 such as salmon, sardines, herring, mackerel, or trout
- Fresh, Frozen, or canned fish or seafood without added sugar or salt

Instructions for Servings:

At least 1 or 3 servings per week

- Have 100 grams (3.5 ounces) of fish

Dairy and Alternatives

What to Eat liberally:

- Milk, kefir, and yogurt that are low-fat and with little or no added sugar
- Plant-based milk and yogurt such as almond milk, coconut milk, hazelnut milk, coconut yogurt
- Cheese with less than 20 percent milk fat

What to Eat Occasionally:

- Milk
- Plain Greek yogurt
- Cottage cheese and ricotta cheese
- Brie cheese, goat cheese, feta cheese, etc.

What to Eat Rarely or Never:

- High-fat milk, butter, and cream
- Sweetened yogurt
- Ice cream
- All processed cheese

Instructions for Servings:

1 to 3 servings per day, such as

- Have 1 cup milk (1% or skim)
- ¾ cup kefir or low-fat yogurt
- 50 grams (1.5 ounces) cheese (less than 20 percent milkfat)

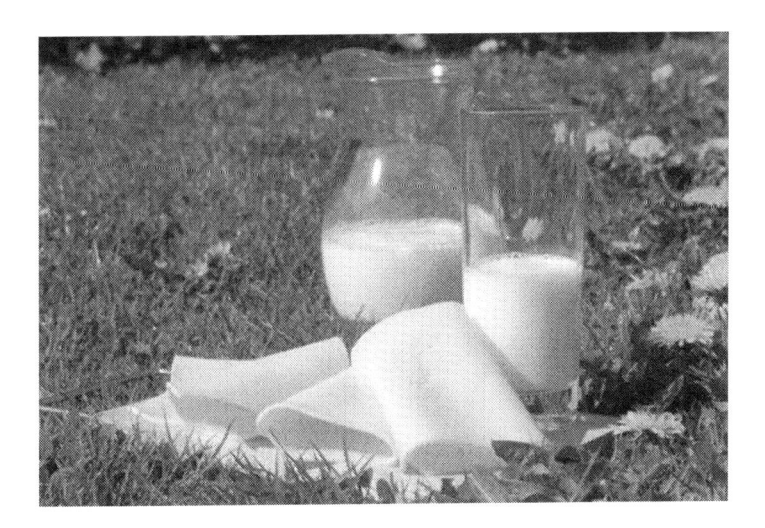

Oil and Fats

What to Eat liberally:

- Avocado and Olives
- Virgin or extra-virgin oil
- Plant-based oil such as coconut oil and avocado oil
- Seeds and nut butter

What to Eat Occasionally:

- Canola oil and soybean oil

What to Eat Rarely or Never:

- Butter
- Trans-fat
- Margarine

Instructions for Servings:

- At least 4 tablespoons or more oil per day at the table or in cooking
- 7 large or 10 small olives per week
- ½ of a medium avocado per week
- 2 tablespoons of seeds and nut butter per week

Sweeteners

What to Eat liberally:

- Consume sweeteners in moderation

What to Eat Occasionally:

- Coconut sugar
- Honey, agave syrup

What to Eat Rarely or Never:

- White sugar

Instructions for Servings:

- 1 to 3 teaspoons per day

Sauces and Condiments

What to Eat liberally:

- Tomato sauce without any sugar
- Pesto sauce, fresh
- Balsamic and apple cider vinegar

What to Eat Occasionally:

- Tzatziki sauce
- Tahini dip
- Aioli

What to Eat Rarely or Never:

- Sweetened sauces such as barbecue sauces
- Teriyaki sauce
- Ketchup

Instructions for Servings:

- 3 to 5 tablespoons per day

Beverages

What to Eat liberally:

- Water
- Green tea and low-fat tea with less sugar
- Coffee with less sugar, decaf coffee

What to Eat Occasionally:

- Red wine
- Other Alcohol

What to Eat Rarely or Never:

- Bottled fruit juices or drinks sweetened with sugar
- Iced tea
- Sweetened coffee
- Soda

Instructions for Servings:

- Women: no more than 2 drinks per day
- Men: no more than 3 drinks per day

1 drink is 5 ounces (142 ml) of drink/wine

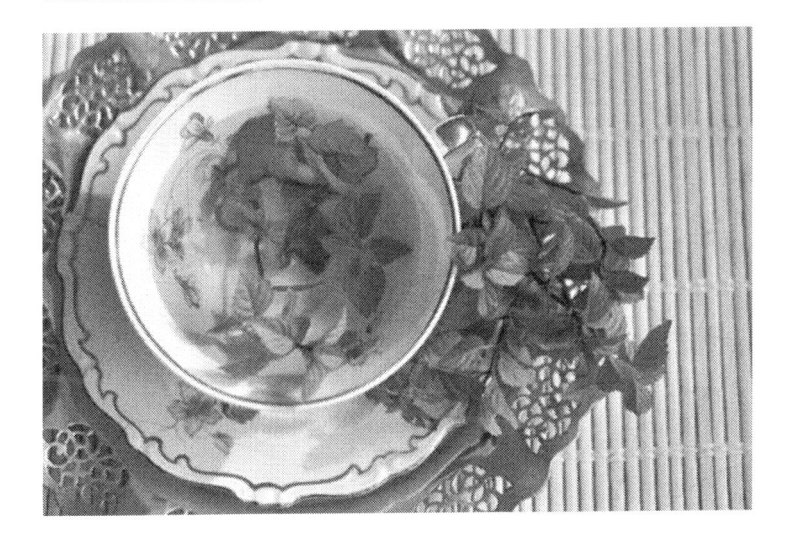

Tips For Success on The Mediterranean Diet

➢ *Eat-In A Way That Is Mindful and Moderate*

The Mediterranean Diet is different from other eating plans because it allows you to have some foods high in fat while still being healthy. Eating this way can also make your brain healthier and help reduce risk factors for heart disease. It is not about starving yourself or cutting out entire food groups; instead, eat moderately without going overboard on certain foods, especially sweets.

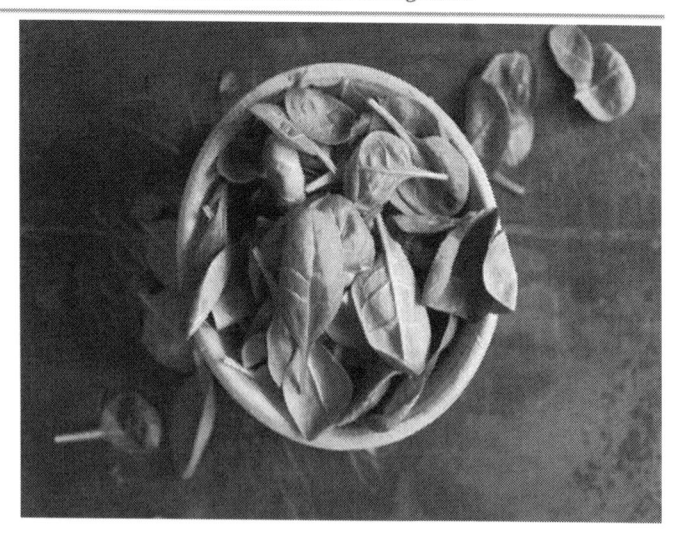

➤ *Find "Gateway" Fruits and Vegetables*

If you do not usually eat a lot of fresh produce, it might be hard to just start eating an apple or broccoli. But there are some vegetables that most people like: gateway vegetables or fruits. You just need to find the one that works for you and start eating that every day. And then, you can gradually go on to other healthy Mediterranean foods like tomatoes, cucumbers, green peppers, and carrots. It might take a year or more before the change happens, but it is worth it because you will feel better. Take it from my experience of losing weight with the Mediterranean diet; this book will help you lose weight in 30 days; however, I would suggest adopting the Mediterranean lifestyle for a year for effective results.

➤ *Include Signature Ingredients*

Tasty food is the best way to make your diet enjoyable. The Mediterranean diet is popular because it has ingredients that everyone likes. You can find recipes from around the Mediterranean that use the same signature ingredients, such as olive oil, whole grains, and vegetables. For protein, use fish, chicken, or a limited amount of red meat. You can create your own collection of Mediterranean dishes. Check out chapter 5 and onwards for inspiration.

> *Incorporate Weight Loss Components*

The Mediterranean diet is not only for weight loss as it is good for keeping the body fit, and healthy but it still plays a major role in weight loss. For effective weight loss, you need to restrict your portions and calories so you can lose some weight. Simple kitchen tools will help with this, like measuring spoons and a food scale. In addition, free apps and websites like myfitnesspal and cronometer will help you figure out how many of the right foods you should eat in a day. It might even make it easier for you to tailor healthy Mediterranean-style meals. A good thumb rule is to plan your meals of 1200 calories or less in total.

> *Treat Meals like a Social Event*

As discussed before, as an important element of the Mediterranean lifestyle, it is common to consider meal times as social events, where all friends and family members get to sit, talk and share laughs. A good human company is all that we need at the end of the day. By adopting a Mediterranean diet, we are going to increase our chances of social freedom and happiness. And, since everyone on the table will be eating the same diet food, this can motivate sticking to the Mediterranean diet for the long run as everyone will understand each other's struggle to live a hearty life. Moreover, you can learn by sharing your experiences with the respective health goals. Even your friend circle could serve as an accountable group to keep a check on each other's diet regime.

> *Eat with Concentration*

We often grab a bite on the go in our fast-paced lives because otherwise, we don't have time. Either we remain immersed in the work or occupied with other professional commitments. With such a lifestyle, we barely get a chance to truly enjoy our meal. But in the Mediterranean regions, people gather on dining tables and keep their phones aside; they truly focus on their food while interacting with other fellows.

> *Exercise is a Must*

For longer positive impacts on your mental and physical health, you need to continue your physical activity. Although any activity involving moving your body is welcome, you can always go for a walk with a friend or family. The reason is that it has been linked with improved heart health, weight loss, and better mental health.

➤ Resist Temptation

It is fairly common to stray away when you are on a diet. For example, you may feel a sudden craving for fried foods like French fries. It is at that point you should remember why you began this journey towards a healthy lifestyle. And, there is always a healthy alternative for your craving, for example, roasted sweet potato fries. Also, always keep healthy snacks within your reach. Munching these nutritious snacks will not only help you resist temptation but also keep you motivated and consistent.

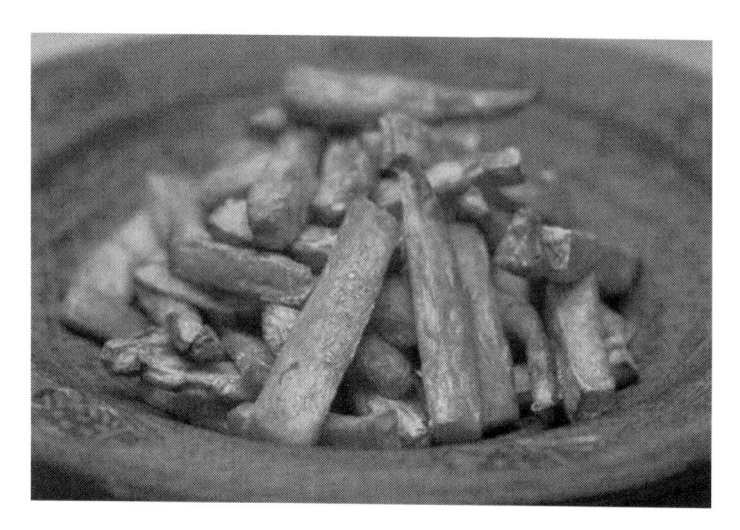

➤ Do not Overwhelm Yourself

When we start something new, our energy levels are always at a peak, but our motivation starts to wear down with time. This is normal because it is okay to fail first when you abandon your decade-old unhealthy eating habits. But you should remind yourself that your older self will thank you for trying so hard to keep your body healthy.

Chapter 4

What to look out for in your Mediterranean Diet

Eating Out on The Mediterranean Diet

The Mediterranean diet is an easy-breezy diet, unlike other diets that limit your food intake and make you starve. This diet offers versatile food options from vegetables to meat. The only restriction it exerts is on the quantity of consumption and style of cooking the food. Our mouths get filled with water at the sight of scrumptious foods, especially if it is at a restaurant, but stopping yourself from eating it just because your diet regime does not permit it, is heartbreaking. No matter the circumstances, sometimes all we want is to eat what our heart desires. The good thing about the Mediterranean diet is the fact that it does not deprive you of any food, as long as it is fresh, organic, and unprocessed.

So, eating out on the Mediterranean diet is easier than you think. The healthier food groups' especially vegetarian food, provide one with enough options to choose from. Ever since the popularity of the Mediterranean diet, many restaurants have updated and modified their menus according to the standards of a Mediterranean diet. Is it not amazing? To be able to eat your favorite food at your favorite eatery without minding calories sure sounds like a dream come true.

Some of the best restaurants for people on the Mediterranean diet could be offering fresh organic farm food and seafood. As the Mediterranean diet is based on the eating habits of Mediterranean countries, so any restaurant serving Italian, Spanish, Greek, or Southern French foods can also compensate for restaurant food cravings. Many vegetarian restaurants serve the best Mediterranean food for you to try. If you happen to notice, a lot of vegetarian restaurants have food options closer to Mediterranean food groups. If you want to satisfy your food cravings while maintaining your diet regime, you must evaluate the frequency of the times you eat out. The reason is that such self-evaluation will assist you in finding a middle ground and help you decide the number of dinners you can afford in a week.

Here are some guidelines you can incorporate in your life and strictly follow when dining out on the Mediterranean diet.

Make Food Choices Based on Overall Diet

You need to ask yourself a simple question to base your food choices surrounding the Mediterranean diet; ask yourself how big part of your diet involves eating out? For example, if you eat once or twice a month, you have nothing to worry about. But if you happen to eat out twice or thrice in a week, then you definitely need to cut it short. Otherwise, there is no point in following the Mediterranean diet.

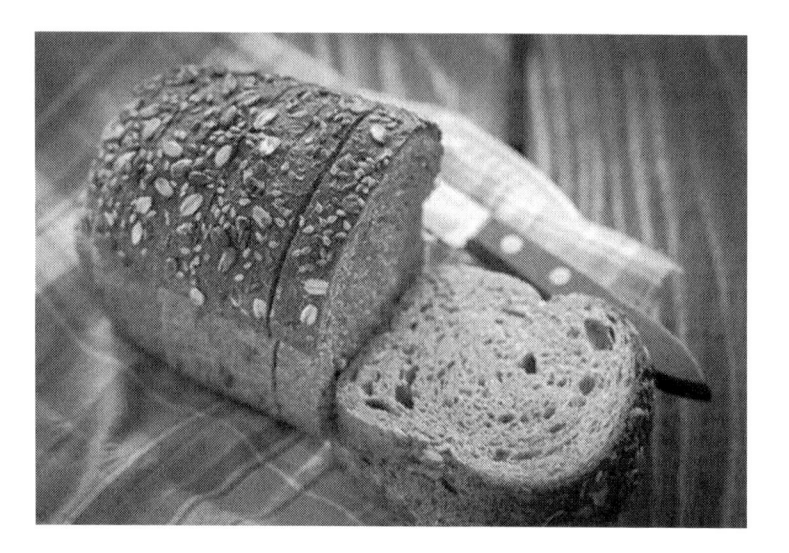

Eat Bread but Mindfully

Although bread is an integral food on a Mediterranean diet, you need to hold your taste buds until the main course is served. By munching on the bread only, you gain substantial calories, minimize your appetite, and deprive yourself of the main meal. This is why the Mediterranean diet preaches minimalism, suggesting that we eat everything healthy but in a limited amount.

Keep A Vegetarian Entrée as A Backup

It is part of human nature to lose interest and feel the urge to give up on a diet regime. Therefore, following and sticking to a diet requires a strong commitment. Still, along the way, you must expect the meltdowns and urges to terminate the Mediterranean regime. It is at this point; vegetarian entrée can save you from succumbing to processed foods. Vegetarian entrées serve plant-based foods containing all the essential nutrients of Mediterranean food, therefore preventing you from giving up the diet and simultaneously satisfying your taste buds.

Look For Boiled and Baked Food on The Menu

You need to securitize the menu thoroughly and look for food that's either boiled or baked. Make sure that the food is sautéed in olive oil instead of butter. Besides that, avoid deep-fried food.

Satisfy Your Craving for Alcoholic Drinks with Wine

Wine is the only alcoholic drink allowed on the Mediterranean diet, with 4-ounce or less per day for women and 8-ounce or less for men.

Always Leave Half Course on The Plate

It may sound unethical and brutal given you are a foodie, but always try to eat half of the food on the plate and then pause for a while. After a few moments, you won't feel as hungry as you were before. This is because it is common for people to go overboard on their cheat meals and throw everything in their stomach, although the hunger could be fulfilled with much less food. Therefore, it is better to eat until half of your stomach is filled, and then, you can get the remaining food parceled and eat the leftovers the next day.

Order Fish Salads

When eating out, try to include fish salad as a side dish beside the main course. Skip the creamy toppings and retreat to the olive oil and vinegar.

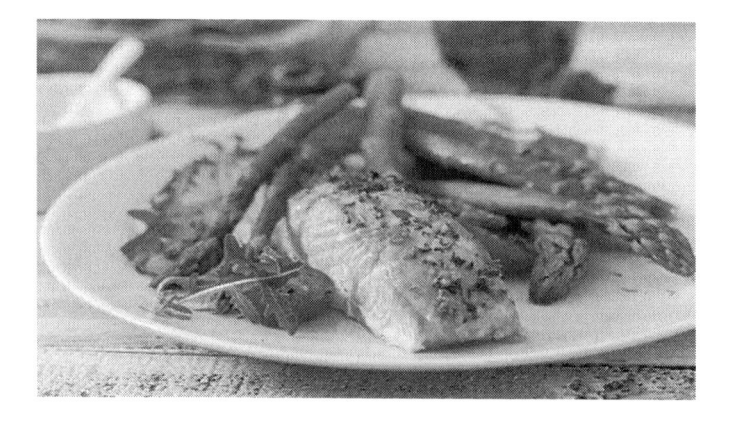

Let The Oil Slide

Most of the time, when we eat out, we do not know what cooking oil is used in the food. To address the latter problem, you can simply try asking the staff if the food is cooked in olive oil or not. If not, then you can either opt for baked dishes or the ones cooked in minimum oil.

Sweet Treats

As far as the desert is concerned, you can skip the scrumptious brownies and pastries and trade them with a plate of fruit salad, cheese, or other low-fat and Mediterranean diet-friendly desserts. The other options for desserts include a slice of chocolate cake or crème Brule.

As discussed in previous chapters, meal times in the Mediterranean diet are considered social events, where everyone gathers at one table and eats together while talking and laughing with one another. This makes dining out at restaurants a natural component of the Mediterranean diet; hence there is no need to stress where and what to eat. You are only required to keep one thing in mind, eat whatever you like but in a controlled amount. Besides that, most of the restaurants make food that is Mediterranean diet-friendly, so you do not have to worry at all.

Now, let's get on to the euphoric experience of Mediterranean-style cooking. In the next section, you will have a meal plan for 30 days. To see the result of the efforts you will put in for weight loss or keep it off, it is important to adopt and follow the Mediterranean diet for a minimum of 30 days. And that's why I have designed meals that give a maximum of 1200 total calories per day as this promotes weight loss. You will find healthy recipes for filling breakfasts, comforting lunches, quick-to-make snacks, hearty dinners, and decadent desserts. And last but not least, some Mediterranean sauces, salad dressings, and dips to maximize the flavors and make your meals extra-tasty!

Feel free to adjust the serving of recipes and experiment with food choices according to your taste and needs.

30 Days Meal Plan

Week 1

Day 1

Breakfast – Greek-Style Frittata (224 calories)

Lunch – Tuna Patties (216 calories)

Snack – Pineapple and Green Smoothie (195 calories)

Dinner – Lentil, Chickpea, and Tomato Soup (291 calories)

Dessert – Coconut, Tahini, and Cashew Bars (155 calories)

Total Calories: 1081 calories

Day 2

Breakfast – Cherry and Walnut Overnight Oats (172 calories)

Lunch – Herby Black Bean Salad with Feta Cheese (245 calories)

Snack – Fish Sticks (238 calories)

Dinner – Grilled Chicken Kabobs (296 calories)

Dessert – Vanilla Baked Pears (216 calories)

Total Calories: 1167 calories

Day 3

Breakfast – Yogurt with Blueberries and Honey (196 calories)

Lunch – Vegetarian Pasta Carbonara (300 calories)

Snack – Orange Salad (186 calories)

Dinner – Italian Minestrone Soup (301.7 calories)

Dessert – Grilled Watermelon Salad (171 calories)

Total Calories: 1154.7 calories

Day 4

Breakfast – Shakshuka (118 calories)

Lunch – Tomato, Basil, and Chickpea Salad (354 calories)

Snack – Trail Mix (218.5 calories)

Dinner – Roasted Tomato and Basil Soup (322 calories)

Dessert – Strawberry Popsicles (38 calories)

Total Calories: 1050.5 calories

Day 5

Breakfast – Greek-Style Frittata (224 calories)

Lunch – Tuna Patties (216 calories)

Snack – Pineapple and Green Smoothie (195 calories)

Dinner – Lentil, Chickpea and Tomato Soup (291 calories)

Dessert – Coconut, Tahini, and Cashew Bars (155 calories)

Total Calories: 1081 calories

Day 6

Breakfast – Cherry and Walnut Overnight Oats (172 calories)

Lunch – Herby Black Bean Salad with Feta Cheese (245 calories)

Snack – Fish Sticks (238 calories)

Dinner – Grilled Chicken Kabobs (296 calories)

Dessert – Vanilla Baked Pears (216 calories)

Total Calories: 1167 calories

Day 7

Breakfast – Yogurt with Blueberries and Honey (196 calories)

Lunch – Vegetarian Pasta Carbonara (300 calories)

Snack – Orange Salad (186 calories)

Dinner – Italian Minestrone Soup (301.7 calories)

Dessert – Grilled Watermelon Salad (171 calories)

Total Calories: 1154.7 calories

Week 2

Day 8

Breakfast – Mini Quiche with Spinach and Mushroom (236 calories)

Lunch – Tabouli Salad (257 calories)

Snack – Chia and Pomegranate Smoothie (208 calories)

Dinner – Cod with Tomatoes and Olives (256 calories)

Dessert – Applesauce Oat Muffins (196 calories)

Total Calories: 1153 calories

Day 9

Breakfast – Quinoa and Chia Oatmeal Mix (162 calories)

Lunch – Mediterranean Cauliflower Pizza (200 calories)

Snack – Kale Chips (176 calories)

Dinner – Greek Turkey Burgers (376 calories)

Dessert – Rice Pudding with Almond Milk (257 calories)

Total Calories: 1171 calories

Day 10

Breakfast – Zucchini with Egg (213 calories)

Lunch – Quinoa and Avocado Salad (236 calories)

Snack – Mediterranean Fruit Salad (201 calories)

Dinner – Greek Pasta (308.3 calories)

Dessert – Watermelon and Mint Granita (168 calories)

Total Calories: 1126.3 calories

Day 11

Breakfast – Breakfast Quinoa with Blueberry and Lemon (269 calories)

Lunch – Mediterranean Salmon (301 calories)

Snack – Tahini and Date Shake (199.4 calories)

Dinner – Shrimp in Garlic Sauce (268.5 calories)

Dessert – Chocolate Dipped Strawberries (235 calories)

Total Calories: 1272.9 calories

Day 12

Breakfast – Mini Quiche with Spinach and Mushroom (236 calories)

Lunch – Tabouli Salad (257 calories)

Snack – Chia and Pomegranate Smoothie (208 calories)

Dinner – Cod with Tomatoes and Olives (256 calories)

Dessert – Applesauce Oat Muffins (196 calories)

Total Calories: 1153 calories

Day 13

Breakfast – Quinoa and Chia Oatmeal Mix (162 calories)

Lunch – Mediterranean Cauliflower Pizza (200 calories)

Snack – Kale Chips (176 calories)

Dinner – Greek Turkey Burgers (376 calories)

Dessert – Rice Pudding with Almond Milk (257 calories)

Total Calories: 1171 calories

Day 14

Breakfast – Zucchini with Egg (213 calories)

Lunch – Quinoa and Avocado Salad (236 calories)

Snack – Mediterranean Fruit Salad (201 calories)

Dinner – Greek Pasta (308.3 calories)

Dessert – Watermelon and Mint Granita (168 calories)

Total Calories: 1126.3 calories

Week 3

Day 15

Breakfast – Spinach and Goat Cheese Quiche (183.1 calories)

Lunch – Chickpea and Quinoa Bowl (273 calories)

Snack – Roasted Chickpeas (208 calories)

Dinner – Hasselback Caprese Chicken (311 calories)

Dessert – Olive Oil Gelato (234 calories)

Total Calories: 1209.1 calories

Day 16

Breakfast – Baked Eggs in Avocado (280 calories)

Lunch – Shrimp Linguine (231 calories)

Snack – Vegetable Chips (100 calories)

Dinner – Greek Red Lentil Soup (293.3 calories)

Dessert – Vanilla Baked Pears (216 calories)

Total Calories: 1120.3 calories

Day 17

Breakfast – Blackberry and Ginger Overnight Bulgur (110 calories)

Lunch – Roasted Eggplants (249.7 calories)

Snack – Flatbread Crackers (190 calories)

Dinner – Grilled Sea Bass (305 calories)

Dessert – Chocolate Avocado Mousse (240 calories)

Total Calories: 1094.7 calories

Day 18

Breakfast – Avocado Toast with Egg (197 calories)

Lunch – Bean Burgers (323.3 calories)

Snack – Baked Zucchini Sticks (132 calories)

Dinner – Sweet and Sour Chicken (375 calories)

Dessert – Baked Apple Slices (228 calories)

Total Calories: 1255.3 calories

Day 19

Breakfast – Spinach and Goat Cheese Quiche (183.1 calories)

Lunch – Chickpea and Quinoa Bowl (273 calories)

Snack – Roasted Chickpeas (208 calories)

Dinner – Hasselback Caprese Chicken (311 calories)

Dessert – Olive Oil Gelato (234 calories)

Total Calories: 1209.1 calories

Day 20

Breakfast – Baked Eggs in Avocado (280 calories)

Lunch – Shrimp Linguine (231 calories)

Snack – Vegetable Chips (100 calories)

Dinner – Greek Red Lentil Soup (293.3 calories)

Dessert – Vanilla Baked Pears (216 calories)

Total Calories: 1120.3 calories

Day 21

Breakfast – Blackberry and Ginger Overnight Bulgur (110 calories)

Lunch – Roasted Eggplants (249.7 calories)

Snack – Flatbread Crackers (190 calories)

Dinner – Grilled Sea Bass (305 calories)

Dessert – Chocolate Avocado Mousse (240 calories)

Total Calories: 1094.7 calories

Week 4

Day 22

Breakfast – Greek-Style Frittata (224 calories)

Lunch – Tuna Patties (216 calories)

Snack – Pineapple and Green Smoothie (195 calories)

Dinner – Lentil, Chickpea and Tomato Soup (291 calories)

Dessert – Coconut, Tahini, and Cashew Bars (155 calories)

Total Calories: 1081 calories

Day 23

Breakfast – Cherry and Walnut Overnight Oats (172 calories)

Lunch – Herby Black Bean Salad with Feta Cheese (245 calories)

Snack – Fish Sticks (238 calories)

Dinner – Grilled Chicken Kabobs (296 calories)

Dessert – Vanilla Baked Pears (216 calories)

Total Calories: 1167 calories

Day 24

Breakfast – Yogurt with Blueberries and Honey (196 calories)

Lunch – Vegetarian Pasta Carbonara (300 calories)

Snack – Orange Salad (186 calories)

Dinner – Italian Minestrone Soup (301.7 calories)

Dessert – Grilled Watermelon Salad (171 calories)

Total Calories: 1154.7 calories

Day 25

Breakfast – Shakshuka (118 calories)

Lunch – Tomato, Basil, and Chickpea Salad (354 calories)

Snack – Trail Mix (218.5 calories)

Dinner – Roasted Tomato and Basil Soup (322 calories)

Dessert – Strawberry Popsicles (38 calories)

Total Calories: 1050.5 calories

Day 26

Breakfast – Greek-Style Frittata (224 calories)

Lunch – Tuna Patties (216 calories)

Snack – Pineapple and Green Smoothie (195 calories)

Dinner – Lentil, Chickpea and Tomato Soup (291 calories)

Dessert – Coconut, Tahini, and Cashew Bars (155 calories)

Total Calories: 1081 calories

Day 27

Breakfast – Cherry and Walnut Overnight Oats (172 calories)

Lunch – Herby Black Bean Salad with Feta Cheese (245 calories)

Snack – Fish Sticks (238 calories)

Dinner – Grilled Chicken Kabobs (296 calories)

Dessert – Vanilla Baked Pears (216 calories)

Total Calories: 1167 calories

Day 28

Breakfast – Yogurt with Blueberries and Honey (196 calories)

Lunch – Vegetarian Pasta Carbonara (300 calories)

Snack – Orange Salad (186 calories)

Dinner – Italian Minestrone Soup (301.7 calories)

Dessert – Grilled Watermelon Salad (171 calories)

Total Calories: 1154.7 calories

Day 29

Breakfast – Mini Quiche with Spinach and Mushroom (236 calories)

Lunch – Tabouli Salad (257 calories)

Snack – Chia and Pomegranate Smoothie (208 calories)

Dinner – Cod with Tomatoes and Olives (256 calories)

Dessert – Applesauce Oat Muffins (196 calories)

Total Calories: 1153 calories

Day 30

Breakfast – Quinoa and Chia Oatmeal Mix (162 calories)

Lunch – Mediterranean Cauliflower Pizza (200 calories)

Snack – Kale Chips (176 calories)

Dinner – Greek Turkey Burgers (376 calories)

Dessert – Rice Pudding with Almond Milk (257 calories)

Total Calories: 1171 calories

Meal Prep Tips

Save time by spending Sunday or any day of the week to prepare the meals for the week ahead. I have always started with making the ingredients lists and checking which foods are present in my pantry and what I need to buy. Meal prep containers for meals, meal prep jars for salad and smoothies, plastic bags, and aluminum foil would greatly help you pack each serving for you and your family members. Some stickers would also be required to label the meals.

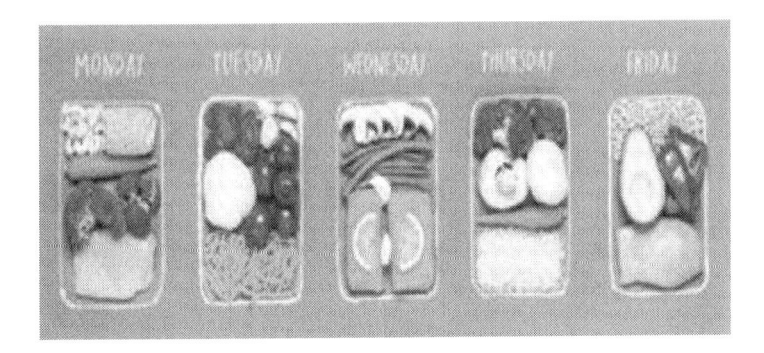

For Meals (breakfast, lunch, snack, dinner, and dessert): When you are done cooking the meals, cool them at room temperature, divide them evenly in meal prep containers and keep them in the refrigerator. When ready to eat, let the meals rest at room temperature for 5 to 10 minutes and then microwave for 1 to 2 minutes at a high heat setting until thoroughly warmed.

You can also pack servings of muffins, frittata, and quiche in just aluminum foil. Prepare oats dishes in the meal prep containers, keep them in the refrigerator and just stir.

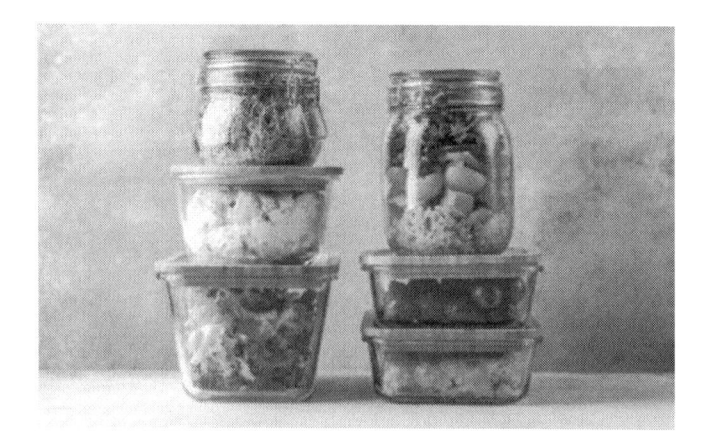

For Salads: Spoon the prepared salad dressing in the bottom of a salad jar, add beans, grains, or hard vegetables such as cucumber, layer with soft vegetables such as avocado and tomatoes, top with proteins, and then layer it with leafy greens of the salad. When ready to eat, mix the salad within the jar until the ingredients have been coated in the salad dressing.

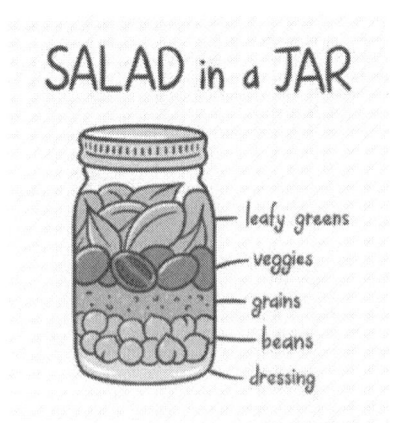

SALAD in a JAR
- leafy greens
- veggies
- grains
- beans
- dressing

For Smoothie:

Add all the solid ingredients in an 8-ounce mason jar or a large plastic bag, seal it, and keep it in the refrigerator until required. When ready to drink, transfer the smoothie ingredients for its bag to a blender, add the liquid and then pulse until smooth. If you have your ingredients in a mason jar, then just pour in the liquid and blend the ingredients with an immersion blender.

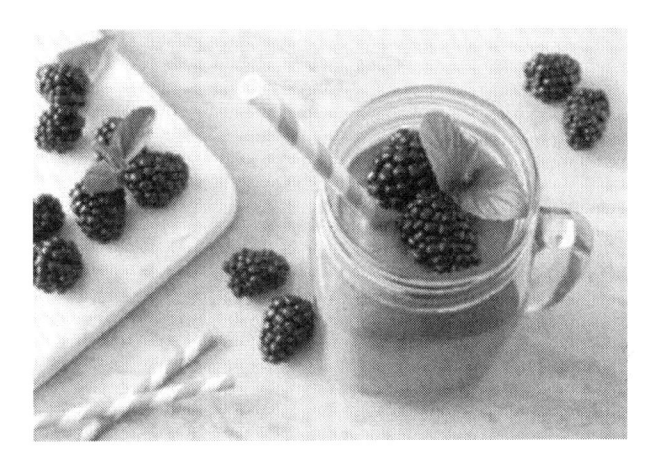

For Sauces, Dips, and Dressings:

Spoon the prepared sauces, dips, and dressing in 4 to 8 ounces mason jars; cover with a thin film of oil to prevent oxidation. Seal the mason jars with their lids and store them in the refrigerator. Try to use sauces, dips, and dressing as fresh and avoid freezing them.

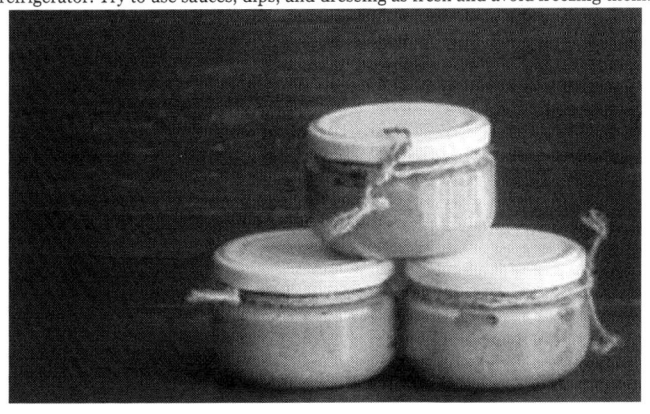

For Snacks:

Like the meal, cool the cooked snacks, divide them in even portions among the meal prep containers or plastic bags, seal them, and keep them in the refrigerator. For snacks such as fruit salad, you can also pack it straight away in the meal prep container. Pack solid snacks such as crackers and chickpeas in a plastic bag.

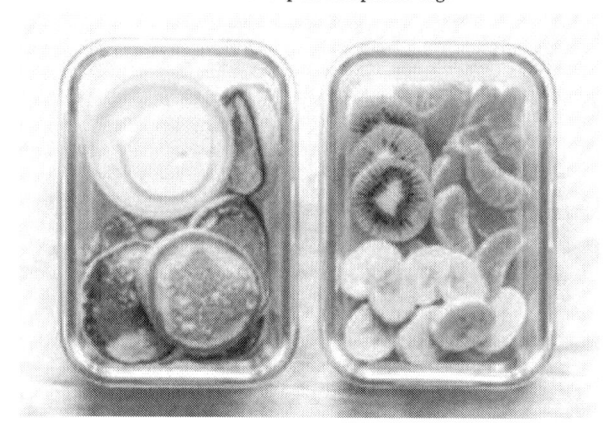

Make sure you label the meal prep containers, jars, and plastic bags with the recipe name and day to eat them.

Chapter 5

Sauces, Dips, and Dressings

Tzatziki Sauce

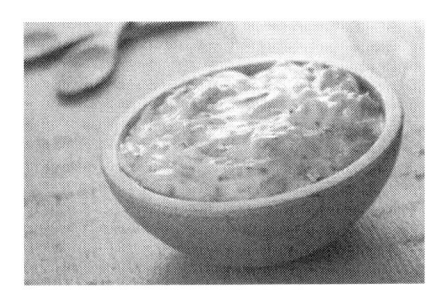

Nutritional Information per Serving

Calories: 28 calories
Fat: 1.9g
Sat. Fat: 0.6g
Carbohydrates: 1.6g
Protein: 0.9g
Fiber: 0.1g

Prep Time: 15 minutes | Cook Time: 0 minutes | Servings: ½ cup; 1 tablespoon per serving

Ingredients

- 1 teaspoon minced garlic
- ½ of a medium cucumber, peeled, grated
- 1/8 teaspoon salt, and more as needed for cucumber
- ¼ teaspoon dried dill
- ¾ tablespoon olive oil
- ½ cup yogurt, low-fat

Directions

- Place the grated cucumber in a colander, sprinkle salt on it, and let it sit for 10 minutes.
- Then squeeze the excess water out from the cucumber, and transfer it to a large bowl.
- Add yogurt, oil, garlic, dill, and ⅛ teaspoon salt, into the bowl, and stir until combined.
- Then cover the bowl with its lid, place it in the refrigerator and let it rest for 30 minutes or more until required and ready to serve.
- Storing Option: For storing the sauce, transfer it to an air-tight container and keep it in the refrigerator for up to 1 week; don't freeze it.

Tahini Sauce

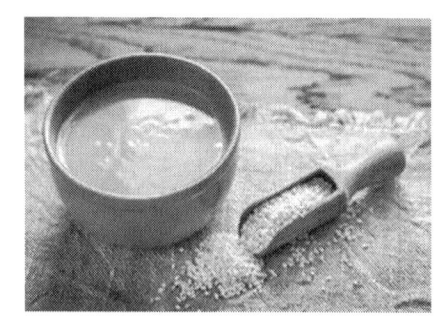

Nutritional Information per Serving

Calories: 124 calories
Fat: 10.8g
Sat. Fat: 1.5g
Carbohydrates: 5.6g
Protein: 3.6g
Fiber: 1.9g

Prep Time: 15 minutes | Cook Time: 0 minutes | Servings: 1 cup; 3 tablespoons per serving

Ingredients

- 4 medium cloves of garlic, peeled, minced
- 1/8 teaspoon ground cumin
- ¼ cup lemon juice
- ½ teaspoon sea salt
- ½ cup tahini
- 6 tablespoons of water, ice-chilled

Directions

- Take a medium bowl, place garlic in it, add lemon juice, stir until well mixed and then let the mixture rest for 10 minutes.
- Take a separate medium bowl, place a fine-mesh sieve on it and then pass the lemon-garlic mixture through it, pressing garlic with the back of a spoon or spatula to extract liquid as much as possible.
- Add tahini into the collected liquid along with cumin and salt, and then whisk. until blended.
- Then whisk 2 tablespoons of water at a time until smooth and creamy sauce comes together, and then store the sauce in an air-tight jar.
- **Storing Option:** Keep the sauce in the refrigerator for up to 1 week or freeze it for up to 1 month.

Pesto Genovese

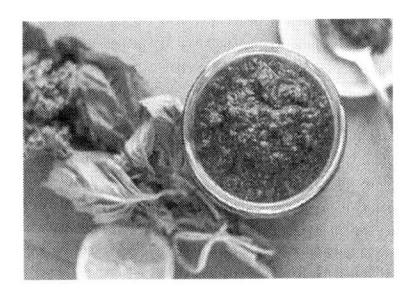

Nutritional Information per Serving

Calories: 123 calories
Fat: 11.5g
Sat. Fat: 3.1g
Carbohydrates: 1.9g
Protein: 3.8g
Fiber: 0.4g

Prep Time: 10 minutes | Cook Time: 0 minutes | Servings: 1 cup; 1 tablespoon per serving

Ingredients

- 2 ounces basil leaves, washed
- 1 clove of garlic, peeled
- 3 tablespoons pine nuts
- ¼ teaspoon salt
- 3 tablespoons Pecorino Sardo cheese, low-fat
- ¼ cup olive oil
- ½ cup parmesan cheese, low-fat

Directions

- Plug in a food processor, add pecorino cheese, parmesan, garlic, pine nuts, salt, and basil leaves.
- Pulse until the mixture turns smooth, and then slowly blend in oil until combined.
- When done, spoon the prepared pesto mixture into a serving bowl, and serve.
- Storing Option: For storing the pesto sauce, transfer it to an air-tight container and keep it in the refrigerator for up to 1 week or freeze it for up to 1 month.

Italian Red Pesto

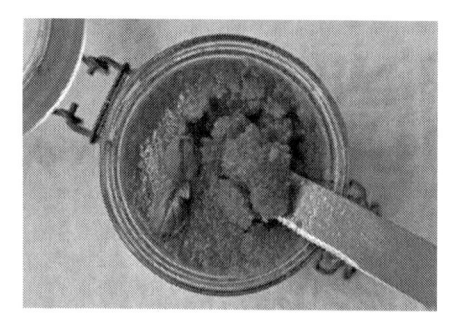

Nutritional Information per Serving

Calories: 91.8 calories
Fat: 8.6g
Sat. Fat: 1.5g
Carbohydrates: 2.06g
Protein: 1.3g
Fiber: 0.5g

Prep Time: 10 minutes | Cook Time: 0 minutes | Servings: ½ cup; 1 tablespoon per serving

Ingredients

- 3 tablespoons almonds
- ½ cup arugula, packed
- ¼ cup sun-dried tomatoes, diced
- 1 clove of garlic, peeled
- 2 tablespoons ricotta cheese, low-fat
- ¼ cup olive oil
- 2 tablespoons grated parmesan cheese, low-fat

Directions

- Plug in a food processor, add garlic, almonds, and tomatoes, and then pulse until chunky.
- Then add arugula, and parmesan, pulse until just mixed, and slowly blend in oil until combined.
- When done, spoon the prepared pesto mixture into a bowl, and serve.

- **Storing Option:** For storing the pesto sauce, transfer it to an air-tight container and keep it in the refrigerator for up to 1 week or freeze it for up to 1 month.

Salsa Verde

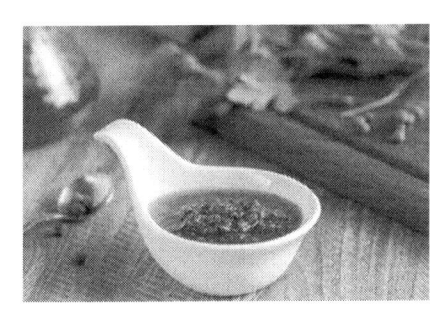

Nutritional Information per Serving

Calories: 48 calories
Fat: 5g
Sat. Fat: 0.7g
Carbohydrates: 0.6g
Protein: 0.6g
Fiber: 0.2g

Prep Time: 10 minutes | Cook Time: 0 minutes | Servings: ½ cup; 1 tablespoon per serving

Ingredients

- ¾ cup parsley, minced
- ½ teaspoon minced garlic
- ¾ tablespoon minced capers
- ¼ teaspoon red chili flakes
- ¼ teaspoon salt
- ¼ teaspoon crushed black pepper
- 3 tablespoons olive oil
- 1 teaspoon lemon juice
- ½ teaspoon lemon zest

Directions

- Take a medium bowl, place parsley in it, add capers and garlic, and stir until mixed.

- Then add lemon zest, lemon juice, salt, red chili flakes, black pepper, and oil, and then stir until mixed and well combined.
- When done, spoon the salsa mixture into a serving bowl, and serve.
- Storing Option: For storing the salsa, transfer it to an air-tight container and keep it in the refrigerator for up to 1 week or freeze it for up to 1 month.

Baba Ganoush

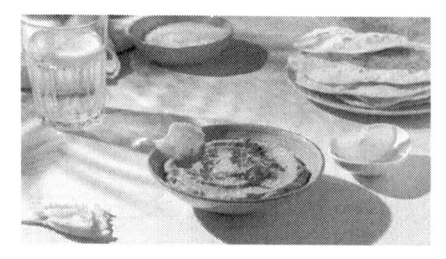

Nutritional Information per Serving

Calories: 27.9 calories
Fat: 1.9g
Sat. Fat: 0.2g
Carbohydrates: 2.2g
Protein: 0.3g
Fiber: 1.1g

Prep Time: 10 minutes | Cook Time: 20 minutes | Servings: 1 cup; 1 tablespoon per serving

Ingredients

- 1 medium eggplant
- 1 clove of garlic, peeled
- ½ teaspoon sumac
- ¼ teaspoon salt
- ¼ teaspoon ground black pepper
- ½ teaspoon cayenne pepper
- 1 ½ tablespoon tahini sauce
- 2 tablespoons olive oil
- 1 tablespoon lemon juice

Directions

- Switch on the oven, then set it to 218 degrees C or 425 degrees F, and preheat.
- Meanwhile, take a baking tray, grease it with cooking spray, and set it aside until required.
- Place the eggplant on a cutting board, slice it in half, and then make a few slits on the skin of the eggplant.
- Sprinkle the eggplant halves with salt, rub it well on the skin of the eggplant, let it sit for 10 minutes, and then wipe it with a cloth dry.
- Place the eggplant skin-side-down on the prepared baking tray, drizzle with oil on top, and then bake for 20 to 30 minutes, or until soft.
- When done, transfer the baked eggplant to a plate, set it aside to cool at room temperature, spoon the insides of the eggplant, and transfer to a food processor.
- Add yogurt, tahini, garlic, lime juice, cayenne, salt, black pepper, and sumac, and pulse until smooth and combined.
- Spoon the dip into a bowl, cover the bowl with its lid, place it into the refrigerator, let it rest for 30 minutes and then serve.
- Storing Option: For storing the baba ganoush, transfer it to an air-tight container and keep it in the refrigerator for up to 5 days; don't freeze it.

Lebanese Hummus

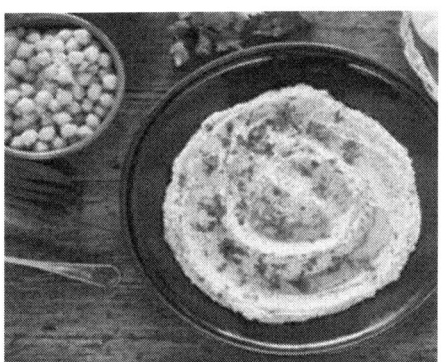

Nutritional Information per Serving

Calories: 152 calories
Fat: 15g
Sat. Fat: 2g
Carbohydrates: 5g
Protein: 2g
Fiber: 1g

Prep Time: 10 minutes | Cook Time: 0 minutes | Servings: 1 cup; 1 tablespoon per serving

Ingredients

- 10 ounces chickpeas, canned, drained, rinsed
- 1 teaspoon minced garlic
- 1 teaspoon crushed pine nuts
- ¼ teaspoon paprika
- 2 tablespoons tahini sauce
- ¼ teaspoon salt
- 2 tablespoons olive oil
- 2 tablespoons lemon juice
- 2 tablespoons water

Directions

- Plug in a food processor, add garlic, chickpeas, paprika, salt, tahini, lemon juice, oil, and water, and pulse until smooth and blended.
- When done, spoon the prepared hummus into a serving bowl, sprinkle pine nuts on top, and serve.
- Storing Option: For storing the hummus, transfer it to an air-tight container and keep it in the refrigerator for up to 1 week or freeze it for up to 1 month.

Guacamole

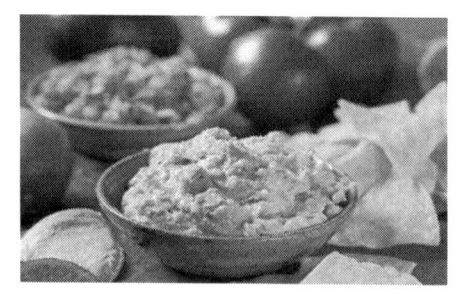

Nutritional Information per Serving

Calories: 44.3 calories
Fat: 2.4g
Sat. Fat: 0.2g
Carbohydrates: 4.4g
Protein: 1.2g
Fiber: 1.1g

Prep Time: 10 minutes | Cook Time: 0 minutes | Servings: 1 cup; 1 tablespoon per serving

Ingredients

- 1 small white onion, peeled, chopped
- 2 medium avocados, halved, pitted
- ½ of a medium tomato, chopped
- ½ of medium green bell pepper, cored, chopped
- 2 tablespoons chopped cilantro, fresh
- ¼ teaspoon salt
- 1 teaspoon olive oil
- 2 tablespoons lemon juice

Directions

- Place the avocados on a cutting board, cut it in half, remove the pit and then spoon the insides of the avocados into a large bowl.
- Take a fork to mash the avocados in the bowl, and then add cilantro, tomato, onion, bell pepper, salt, lemon juice, and oil.
- Stir until combined and well mixed, then spoon the prepared mixture into a serving bowl, and serve.
- Storing Option: For storing the guacamole, spoon it into an air-tight container, smooth the top, cover it with a thin layer of lemon juice, shut the container tightly with its lid, and refrigerate for up to 1 week; don't freeze it.

Roasted Tomato Spread (Matbucha)

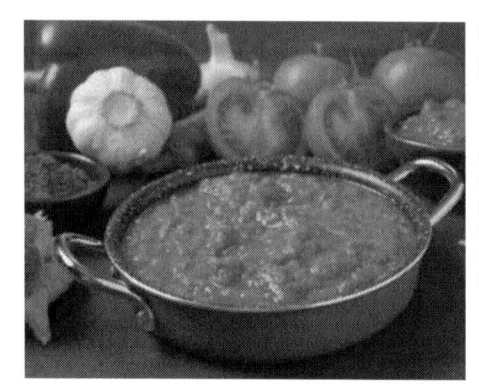

Nutritional Information per Serving

Calories: 27.5 calories
Fat: 1.7g
Sat. Fat: 0.2g
Carbohydrates: 2.6g
Protein: 0.3g
Fiber: 0.7g

Prep Time: 10 minutes | Cook Time: 20 minutes | Servings: 1 cup; 1 tablespoon per serving

Ingredients

- 4 small tomatoes, halved
- 1 large green bell pepper, quartered
- 3 cloves of garlic, peeled
- 2 tablespoons cilantro leaves
- 1 large white onion, peeled, quartered
- 2 tablespoons parsley leaves
- ¼ teaspoon salt
- 1 teaspoon red chili flakes
- ¼ teaspoon ground black pepper
- 1 tablespoon lemon juice
- 2 tablespoons olive oil, divided

Directions

- Switch on the oven, then set it to 190 degrees C or 347 degrees F, and preheat.
- Meanwhile, take a baking tray, grease it with cooking spray, and set it aside.

- Take a large bowl, place tomatoes, green peppers, onions, and garlic in it, add 1 tablespoon oil, salt, red pepper flakes, and black pepper, and toss until well mixed.
- Transfer the vegetables to the prepared baking tray and spread them in a single layer.
- Place the tray in the oven and bake for 20 to 30 minutes, or until golden brown.
- When done, let the vegetables cool at room temperature and then transfer them into a food processor.
- Add remaining oil along with parsley and cilantro, pulse until the mixture is combined and chunky, spoon the dip into a bowl and then serve.
- Storing Option: For storing the spread, transfer it to an air-tight container and keep it in the refrigerator for up to 1 week or freeze it for up to 1 month.

Pickled Mango Sauce

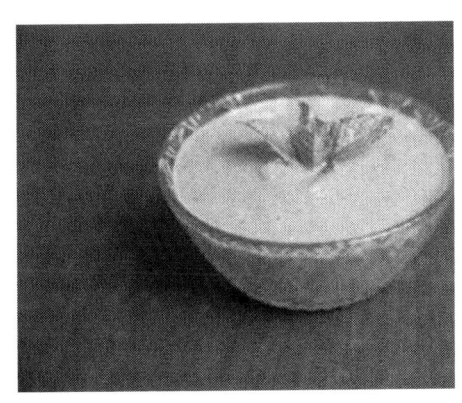

Nutritional Information per Serving

Calories: 27.8 calories
Fat: 1.7g
Sat. Fat: 0.2g
Carbohydrates: 2.7g
Protein: 0.2g
Fiber: 0.4g

Prep Time: 15 minutes | Cook Time: 8 minutes | Servings: 1 ½ cups; 1 tablespoon per serving

Ingredients

- 1 large mango, peeled, cut into chunks
- ½ teaspoon minced garlic
- 1 tablespoon coconut sugar
- ¾ tablespoon salt
- ½ teaspoon mustard seeds
- ½ teaspoon ground fenugreek
- 1 teaspoon cumin seeds
- ½ teaspoon ground coriander
- ½ teaspoon turmeric powder
- ½ teaspoon ground black pepper
- 1 tablespoon paprika
- 3 tablespoons olive oil
- ½ cup water

Directions

- Place the mango chunks on a cutting board, sprinkle with salt, transfer into a glass jar, close with its lid and let the jar rest in the sun for 5 days.
- Then drain the excess water out from the jar, spread the mango chunks on parchment paper, and let them dry for 4 hours.
- Take a small pot, place it over low heat, add mustard seed, fenugreek, cumin, coriander, turmeric, black pepper, paprika.
- Stir while cooking for 3 minutes, add coconut sugar and garlic, cook for 3 minutes, add mangoes and water and then stir until well combined.
- Then plug in a blender, add the prepared mango mixture, pulse until smooth, and serve.
- **Storing Option:** For storing the sauce, transfer it to an air-tight container and keep it in the refrigerator for up to 1 week; don't freeze it.

Cherry Tomato Sauce

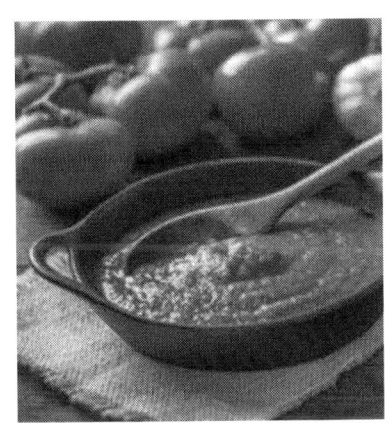

Nutritional Information per Serving

Calories: 21 calories
Fat: 1.7g
Sat. Fat: 0.2g
Carbohydrates: 1.1g
Protein: 0.2g
Fiber: 0.2g

Prep Time: 10 minutes | Cook Time: 20 minutes | Servings: 2 cups; 1 tablespoon per serving

Ingredients

- 1 quart of cherry tomatoes, stems removed
- 1 teaspoon minced garlic
- ½ teaspoon dried oregano
- ¼ teaspoon salt
- ¼ teaspoon ground black pepper
- ¼ cup olive oil
- 2 tablespoons balsamic vinegar

Directions

- Switch on the oven, then set it to 204 degrees C or 400 degrees F, and preheat.

- Meanwhile, take a baking tray, grease it with cooking spray, and set it aside until required.
- Scatter the cherry tomatoes on the prepared baking tray in a single layer, drizzle with oil and balsamic vinegar, and then sprinkle salt, black pepper, oregano, and garlic.
- Bake the tomatoes for 20 minutes, or until soft, let the tomatoes cool at room temperature and transfer into a blender.
- Pulse the tomato mixture until smooth, and then serve.
- Storing Option: For storing the sauce, transfer it to an air-tight container and keep it in the refrigerator for up to 1 week or freeze it for up to 1 month.

Roasted Red Pepper Dip (Muhammara)

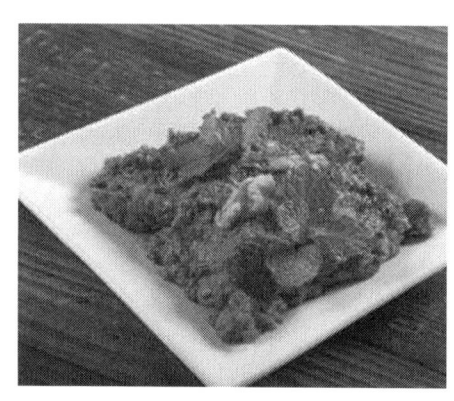

Nutritional Information per Serving

Calories: 54 calories
Fat: 4.7g
Sat. Fat: 0.6g
Carbohydrates: 2.1g
Protein: 0.6g
Fiber: 0.4g

Prep Time: 10 minutes | Cook Time: 20 minutes | Servings: 1 cup; 1 tablespoon per serving

Ingredients

- ½ cup walnuts, roasted
- 1 medium bell pepper, halved,
- ¼ teaspoon crushed red pepper flakes

- roasted
- 1 clove of garlic, peeled
- 2 tablespoons whole-wheat breadcrumbs
- ½ teaspoon salt
- ½ teaspoon ground cumin
- 3 tablespoons olive oil
- ½ teaspoon pomegranate molasses
- ½ tablespoon lemon juice

Directions

- Plug in a blender, add roasted bell pepper, roasted walnuts, oil, salt, cumin, red pepper, and breadcrumbs.
- Add garlic, molasses, and lemon juice, pulse until smooth and well combined.
- When done, spoon the prepared mixture into a serving bowl, and serve.
- Storing Option: For storing the dip, transfer it to an air-tight container and keep it in the refrigerator for up to 1 week; don't freeze it.

Ranch Dressing

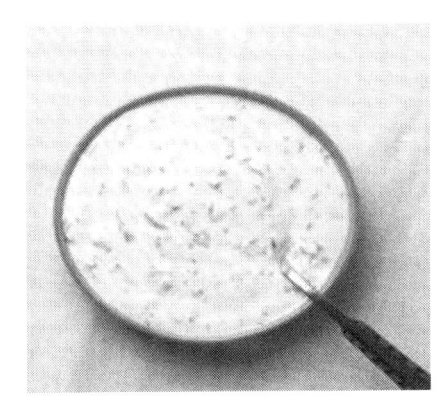

Nutritional Information per Serving

Calories: 52.7 calories
Fat: 5.5g
Sat. Fat: 0.9g
Carbohydrates: 0.9g
Protein: 0.4g
Fiber: 0.01g

Prep Time: 10 minutes | Cook Time: 10 minutes | Servings: 1 cup; 1 tablespoon per serving

Ingredients

- ½ tablespoon parsley
- ½ tablespoon dill
- ½ tablespoon onion powder
- ½ tablespoon garlic powder
- ¼ teaspoon salt
- ¼ teaspoon ground black pepper
- ½ tablespoon apple cider vinegar
- ¼ cup yogurt, low-fat
- ½ cup mayonnaise, low-fat

Directions

- Take a large mixing bowl, place mayonnaise, yogurt, and vinegar in it, and whisk until well combined.
- Add onion powder, garlic powder, salt, black pepper, dill, parsley, and whisk until well mixed and smooth.
- When done, spoon the prepared dressing into a serving bowl, and serve.
- Storing Option: For storing the dressing, transfer it to an air-tight container and keep it in the refrigerator for up to 5 days; don't freeze it.

Tangy Italian Salad Dressing

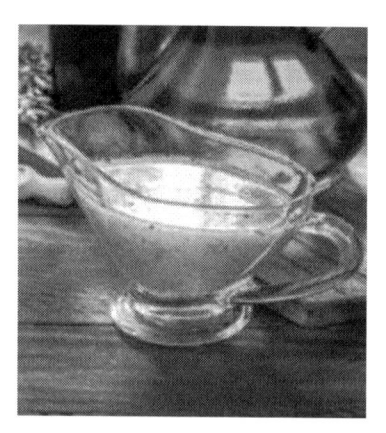

Nutritional Information per Serving

Calories: 81.1 calories
Fat: 8.5g
Sat. Fat: 1.2g
Carbohydrates: 0.6g
Protein: 0.6g
Fiber: 0.6g

Prep Time: 5 minutes | Cook Time: 0 minutes | Servings: ½ cup; 1 tablespoon per serving

Ingredients

- 1 teaspoon minced garlic
- ¼ teaspoon dried oregano
- ¼ teaspoon dried basil
- ¼ teaspoon salt
- ½ cup olive oil
- ¼ teaspoon whole-grain mustard
- 3 tablespoons red wine vinegar
- 1 tablespoon lemon juice

Directions

- Take a large jar, add garlic, basil, oregano, salt, and add mustard, oil, vinegar, and lemon juice.
- Cover the jar with its lid and then shake it well until combined and mixed.
- When done, spoon the prepared dressing into a serving bowl, and serve.
- Storing Option: For storing the dressing, transfer it to an air-tight container and keep it in the refrigerator for up to 5 days; don't freeze it.

Yogurt Tahini Dressing

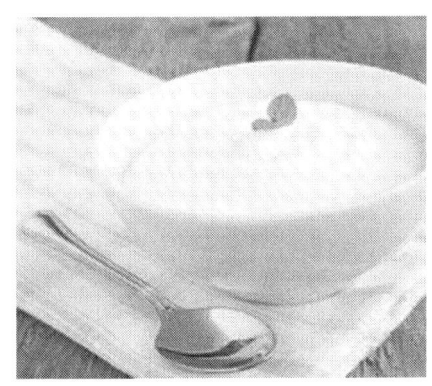

Nutritional Information per Serving

Calories: 27 calories
Fat: 1.5g
Sat. Fat: 0.7g
Carbohydrates: 1.8g
Protein: 1.3g
Fiber: 0.1g

Prep Time: 5 minutes | Cook Time: 0 minutes | Servings: 1 cup; 1 tablespoon per serving

Ingredients

- ½ teaspoon minced garlic
- ¼ teaspoon salt
- 2 tablespoons lemon juice
- 2 teaspoons tahini
- 1 cup yogurt, low-fat
- ½ teaspoon lemon zest

Directions

- Take a medium bowl, place yogurt and tahini in it, add salt, garlic, lemon juice, and lemon zest, and stir until well combined.
- When done, spoon the prepared dressing into a serving bowl, and serve.
- Storing Option: For storing the dressing, transfer it to an air-tight container and keep it in the refrigerator for up to 5 days; don't freeze it.

Balsamic, Dill and Yogurt Dressing

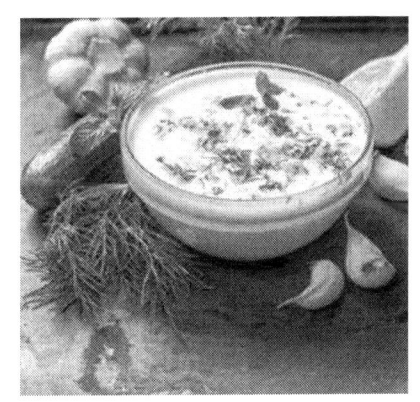

Nutritional Information per Serving

Calories: 67 calories
Fat: 6.9g
Sat. Fat: 1.1g
Carbohydrates: 0.5g
Protein: 0.5g
Fiber: 0.05g

Prep Time: 5 minutes | Cook Time: 0 minutes | Servings: ½ cup; 1 tablespoon per serving

Ingredients

- 1 teaspoon minced garlic
- ¼ teaspoon salt
- ¼ teaspoon dried oregano
- ¼ teaspoon dried dill
- ¼ cup olive oil
- ½ tablespoon whole-grain mustard
- ¼ cup yogurt, low-fat
- 2 tablespoons apple cider vinegar

Directions

- Take a medium bowl, place garlic, yogurt, and vinegar in it, add salt, oregano, dill, mustard, and whisk until well combined.
- Then gently whisk in oil until incorporated, and smooth, and then serve.
- **Storing Option:** For storing the dressing, transfer it to an air-tight container and keep it in the refrigerator for up to 5 days; don't freeze it.

Chapter 6

Breakfast

Greek-Style Frittata

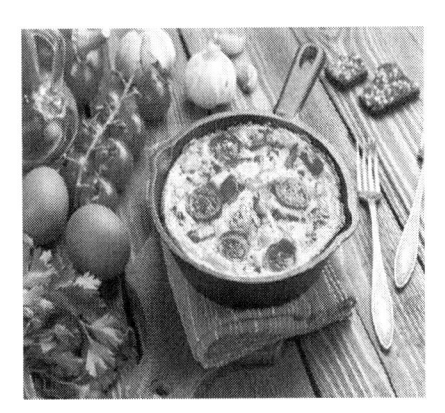

Nutritional Information per Serving

Calories: 224 calories
Fat: 15g
Sat. Fat: 4g
Carbohydrates: 7g
Protein: 15g
Fiber: 2g

Prep Time: 10 minutes | Cook Time: 12 minutes | Servings: 1 Frittata, 1 slice per serving

Ingredients

- ½ cup dried tomato slices, not oil-packed
- 6 tablespoons Italian marinated olive antipasto
- 1 teaspoon dried oregano, crushed
- 8 large eggs, at room temperature
- 2 tablespoons olive oil
- ½ cup boiling water
- 4 tablespoons crumbled feta cheese, reduced-fat

- ½ cup roasted red sweet peppers, chopped
- ¼ teaspoon ground black pepper
- 1 tablespoon chopped oregano

Directions

- Switch on the oven, then set it to 425 degrees F and let it preheat.
- Meanwhile, take a small bowl, place dried tomatoes in it, pour in the boiling water, stir until just mixed and let the tomatoes stand for 5 minutes.
- In the meantime, take a large bowl, crack eggs in it and then whisk until blended.
- Add dried oregano, red pepper, olive antipasto, and cheese and stir until just mixed.
- Drain the soaked tomatoes, reserving their liquid, and then stir this liquid into the prepared egg mixture.
- Take a large heat-proof skillet pan, place it over medium heat, add oil, and when hot, pour in the egg mixture and then spread it evenly.
- Scatter the soak tomato slices on top, cook for 3 to 4 minutes until the bottom begins to set, and then transfer the skillet pan into the oven.
- Continue cooking the frittata for 5 to 8 minutes until thoroughly cooked and top turn golden.
- When done, slide the frittata into a plate, let it rest for 5 minutes and then cut it into four slices.
- Sprinkle chopped oregano over the frittata slices and then serve.

Spinach and Goat Cheese Quiche

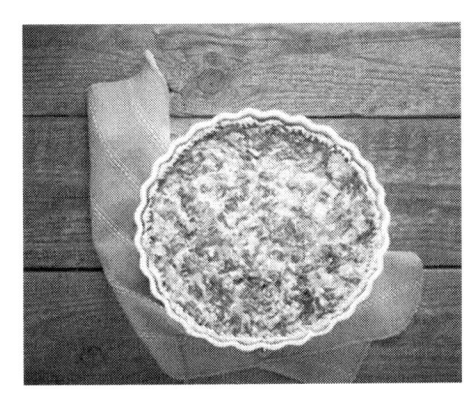

Nutritional Information per Serving

Calories: 183.1 calories
Fat: 10.7g
Sat. Fat: 4.1g
Carbohydrates: 13g
Protein: 9.8g
Fiber: 0.8g

Prep Time: 10 minutes | Cook Time: 30 minutes | Servings: 1 Quiche, 1 slice per serving

Ingredients

- 6 ounces spinach leaves, fresh, chopped
- 1 frozen pie crust, whole-grain, thawed
- 2 medium eggs, at room temperature
- ¼ teaspoon salt
- 1/3 cup half-and-half
- ¼ teaspoon ground black pepper
- 4 slices of goat cheese, fresh, low-fat
- ¼ cup water
- 2 tablespoons sour cream, low-fat

Directions

- Switch on the oven, then set it to 390 degrees F and let it preheat.
- Meanwhile, take a medium skillet pan, place it over medium heat, pour in the water, and then bring it to a simmer.

- Add spinach leaves, cook them for 3 to 4 minutes until leaves have wilted, drain them and then squeeze well to remove excess water.
- Take a medium bowl, crack eggs in it, whisk until blended and then whisk in salt, half-and-half, black pepper, and sour cream until smooth.
- Add the cooked spinach into the egg mixture and then stir until just mixed.
- Place the pie crust into a greased pie pan, fill it with the prepared egg mixture, smooth the top and then scatter the goat cheese slices on top.
- Place the prepared pie pan into the oven and then bake for 20 to 30 minutes until the quiche has set and the top turns golden brown.
- When done, let the quiche in its pan for 5 minutes, then transfer it to a cutting board, cut it into four slices and serve.

Mini Quiche with Spinach and Mushroom

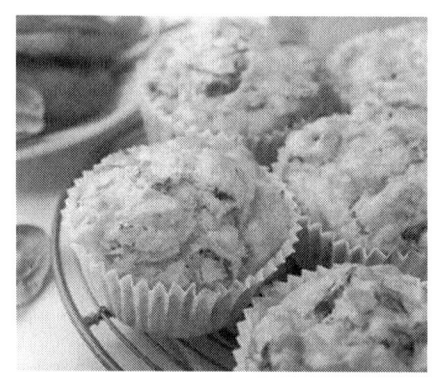

Nutritional Information per Serving

Calories: 236 calories
Fat: 16.4g
Sat. Fat: 5.8g
Carbohydrates: 7.1g
Protein: 15.5g
Fiber: 1.5g

Prep Time: 10 minutes | Cook Time: 30 minutes | Servings: 6 mini-quiche; 2 quiches per serving

Ingredients

- 2 ounces spinach leaves, fresh, chopped
- 4 ounces shiitake mushrooms, sliced
- ½ cup sliced white onion
- ½ tablespoon minced garlic
- 1 teaspoon minced thyme
- ¼ teaspoon salt
- 1 teaspoon whole-grain mustard
- ¼ teaspoon ground black pepper
- 1 tablespoon olive oil
- 4 medium eggs, at room temperature
- 6 tablespoons coconut milk, unsweetened, low-fat
- 6 tablespoons shredded Gruyere or parmesan cheese, low-fat

Directions

- Switch on the oven, then set it to 325 degrees F and let it preheat.
- Meanwhile, take a medium skillet pan, place it over medium heat, add oil and when hot, add mushrooms.
- Spread the mushrooms in a single layer and then cook for 4 minutes per side until brown.
- Then add onion, cook for 2 minutes until softened, stir in garlic and thyme and continue cooking for 2 minutes.
- Add spinach, stir until just mixed, cook for 2 minutes and then remove the pan from heat.
- Take a medium bowl, crack the eggs in it, add salt, black pepper, and mustard, pour in the mustard, and then whisk until blended.
- Add the mushroom mixture along with cheese and then stir until just mixed.
- Take 6 silicone muffin cups, grease them with oil, evenly fill them with the prepared mushroom mixture and then bake for 15 to 20 minutes until thoroughly cooked and firm.
- When done, let the quiche rest in the muffin cups for 5 minutes and then serve.

Baked Eggs in Avocado

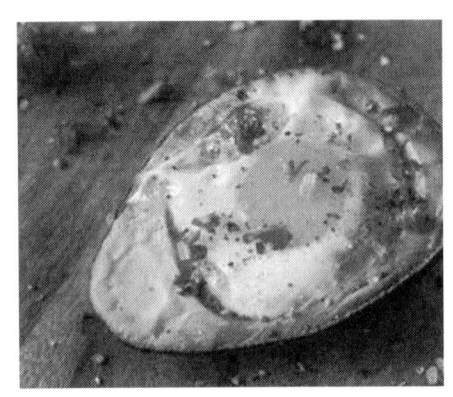

Nutritional Information per Serving

Calories: 280 calories
Fat: 23.5g
Sat. Fat: 4.9g
Carbohydrates: 9.3g
Protein: 11.3g
Fiber: 6.9g

Prep Time: 10 minutes | Cook Time: 15 minutes | Servings: 2; 1 avocado half per serving

Ingredients

- 1 avocado, halved, pitted
- 2 teaspoons chopped chives, fresh
- ¼ teaspoon sea salt
- ¼ teaspoon dried parsley
- ¼ teaspoon ground black pepper
- 2 small eggs, at room temperature

Directions

- Switch on the oven, then set it to 425 degrees F and let it preheat.
- Meanwhile, take a medium bowl and crack the eggs in it, keeping the yolk intact.
- Take a baking dish, arrange avocado halves in it cut-side-up and then spoon an egg yolk into each half.

- Then divide the egg white evenly between the avocado halves and then season with salt, black pepper, chives, and parsley.
- Place the prepared baking dish containing avocado halves into the oven and then bake for 15 minutes or until the eggs have cooked to the desired level.
- Serve straight away.

Avocado Toast with Egg

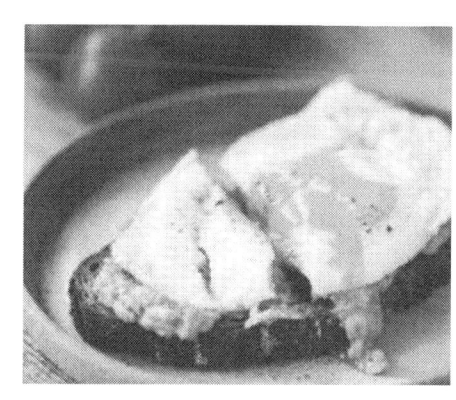

Nutritional Information per Serving

Calories: 197 calories
Fat: 17g
Sat. Fat: 6g
Carbohydrates: 5g
Protein: 7g
Fiber: 3g

Prep Time: 10 minutes | Cook Time: 10 minutes | Servings: 4; 1 toast per serving

Ingredients

- 4 slices of whole-wheat bread
- 1 avocado, peeled, pitted, sliced
- ¼ teaspoon sea salt
- 4 tablespoons butter, low-fat
- ¼ teaspoon ground black pepper
- 4 eggs, at room temperature

Directions

- Prepare the bread slices and for this, toast them until golden and crispy to the desired level.

- Meanwhile, take a medium bowl, place avocado slices in it and then mash with a fork.
- Fry the egg, and for this, take a medium skillet pan, place it over medium heat, add 1 tablespoon butter and when it melts, crack the egg in it and then cook for 5 to 7 minutes until cooked to the desired level.
- Assemble the toast and for this, spread ¼ of the mashed avocado over the toast, sprinkle some salt and black pepper over the top and then top with a fried egg.
- Serve straight away.

Zucchini with Egg

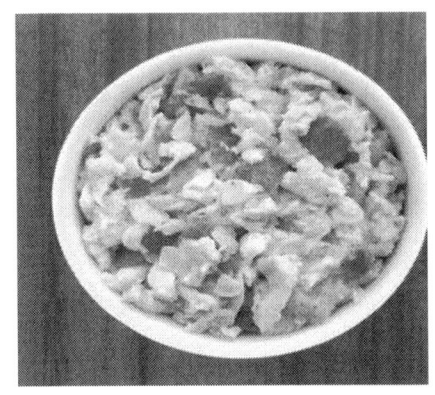

Nutritional Information per Serving

Calories: 213 calories
Fat: 15.7g
Sat. Fat: 3.1g
Carbohydrates: 11.2g
Protein: 10.2g
Fiber: 3.6g

Prep Time: 5 minutes | Cook Time: 18 minutes | Servings: 2; 1 plate per serving

Ingredients

- 2 large zucchinis, ends trimmed, diced
- ½ teaspoon salt
- 1 ½ tablespoon olive oil
- ¼ teaspoon ground black pepper
- 1 teaspoon water
- 2 large eggs, at room

temperature

Directions

- Take a medium skillet pan, place it over medium-high heat, add oil and when hot, add zucchini and then cook for 10 minutes until tender.
- Stir salt and black pepper into the zucchini and continue cooking for 1 minute.
- Take a medium bowl, crack the eggs in it, add water and then whisk until blended.
- Pour the blended eggs over the cooked zucchini and then cook for 5 minutes until eggs have scrambled to the desired level.
- Taste the scrambled eggs to adjust seasonings, divide evenly between two plates, and then serve.

Shakshuka

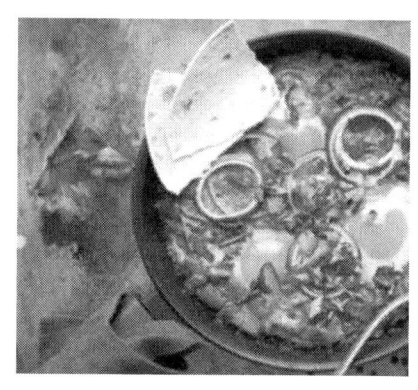

Nutritional Information per Serving

Calories: 118 calories
Fat: 9g
Sat. Fat: 2g
Carbohydrates: 4g
Protein: 7g
Fiber: 1g

Prep Time: 5 minutes | Cook Time: 18 minutes | Servings: 4; 1 egg with tomato mixture per serving

Ingredients

- ½ medium white onion, peeled, chopped
- ½-pound tomatoes, halved
- ¼ cup baby spinach, chopped
- ¼ teaspoon minced garlic
- ¼ teaspoon salt
- 1 tablespoon olive oil
- ¼ teaspoon ground pepper
- ½ teaspoon ground cumin
- 4 large eggs, at room temperature

Directions

- Switch on the oven, then set it to 400 degrees F and let it preheat.
- Meanwhile, take a large heat-proof skillet pan, place it over medium-high heat, add oil, and when hot, add onion and then cook for 4 minutes until golden brown.
- Add salt, black pepper, cumin, and garlic, stir until mixed, and then continue cooking for 1 minute.
- Add tomato halves, stir until just mixed, then transfer the pan into the oven and continue cooking for 5 minutes until tomatoes have roasted.
- When done, stir the tomatoes well, make four small spaces in the tomato mixture and then carefully crack an egg into each space.
- Return the pan into the oven and continue cooking for 3 to 5 minutes until egg yolks turn runny.
- When done, sprinkle spinach over the eggs and then serve with toasted slices of whole-wheat baguette.

Cherry and Walnut Overnight Oats

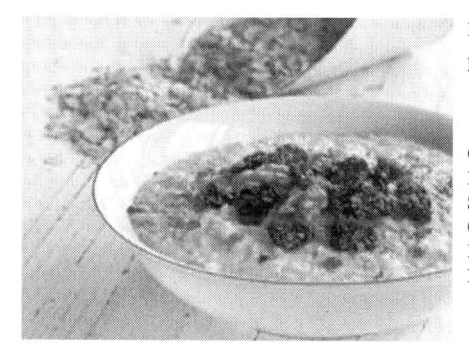

Nutritional Information per Serving

Calories: 162 calories
Fat: 6.2g
Sat. Fat: 1.8g
Carbohydrates: 23g
Protein: 4.3g
Fiber: 2.5g

Prep Time: 8 hours and 10 minutes | Cook Time: 0 minutes | Servings: 4; 1 bowl per serving

Ingredients

- 1 cup rolled oats, old-fashioned
- 2 tablespoons chopped dried cherries
- ½ teaspoon salt
- 4 teaspoons coconut sugar
- 1 cup water
- 2 tablespoons toasted chopped walnuts
- 1 teaspoon lemon zest
- 4 tablespoons reduced-fat cream cheese

Directions

- Take a large bowl, place oats in it, add salt, pour in the water, and then stir until combined.

- Cover the bowl with its lid, place it in the refrigerator and then let the oats rest for a minimum of 8 hours or overnight.
- When ready to eat, bring oats to room temperature, stir until just mixed, and then divide evenly among four bowls.
- Sprinkle with sugar, top with cheese, walnuts, and cream cheese, sprinkle with lemon zest and then serve.

Blackberry and Ginger Overnight Bulgur

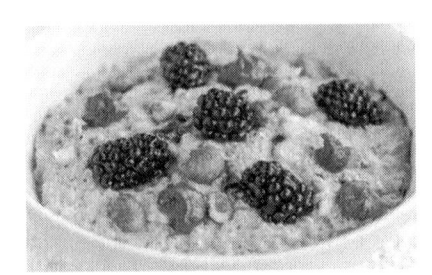

Nutritional Information per Serving

Calories: 110 calories
Fat: 1g
Sat. Fat: 0.5g
Carbohydrates: 22.5g
Protein: 4g
Fiber: 1.5g

Prep Time: 8 hours and 10 minutes | Cook Time: 0 minutes | Servings: 4; 1 bowl per serving

Ingredients

- 1 cup bulgur
- 8 tablespoons honey, organic
- 1 cup blackberries, fresh
- 1 teaspoon ground ginger
- 1 1/3 cup coconut yogurt, low-fat
- 12 tablespoons coconut milk, unsweetened, low-fat

Directions

- Take a large bowl, place bulgur in it, add honey and ginger, and then pour in the milk and yogurt.

- Stir until well combined, cover the bowl with its lid, place it in the refrigerator and then let the bulgur rest for a minimum of 8 hours or overnight.
- When ready to eat, bring bulgur to room temperature, stir until just mixed, and then divide evenly among four bowls.
- Top the bulgur with the blackberries and then serve.

Quinoa and Chia Oatmeal Mix

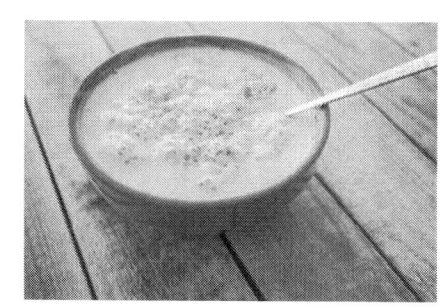

Nutritional Information per Serving

Calories: 172 calories
Fat: 3.2g
Sat. Fat: 0.5g
Carbohydrates: 28g
Protein: 5.2g
Fiber: 4.1g

Prep Time: 10 minutes | Cook Time: 15 minutes | Servings: 4; 1 bowl per serving

Ingredients

For the Oatmeal Mix:

- 1 cup rolled oats, old fashioned
- ½ cup dried fruit mixture
- ½ cup rolled wheat
- ¼ cup chia seeds
- ½ cup quinoa
- ¼ teaspoon salt
- ½ teaspoon ground cinnamon

For Each Serving:

- ½ tablespoon chopped walnuts
- 1 tablespoon honey, raw
- ½ tablespoon sliced almonds
- 1 cup almond milk, unsweetened, low-fat

Directions

- Prepare the mix and for this, take a large bowl, place oats in it, and then add dried fruit mix, wheat, chia seeds, and quinoa.
- Add salt and cinnamon, stir until well mixed, and then store it by transferring the mixture into an air-tight container.
- When ready to eat, take a small saucepan, place it over medium heat, add ¼ cup of the oatmeal mix and 1 cup milk and then bring the mixture to a boil.
- Then switch heat to low level and simmer the oatmeal for 10 to 15 minutes until thickened to the desired level, covering the pan partially.
- When done, remove the pan from heat, cover the pan with a lid and let the mixture stand for 5 minutes.
- Transfer the oatmeal mixture into a bowl, drizzle with honey, sprinkle walnuts and almonds on top, and then serve.

Quinoa with Blueberry and Lemon

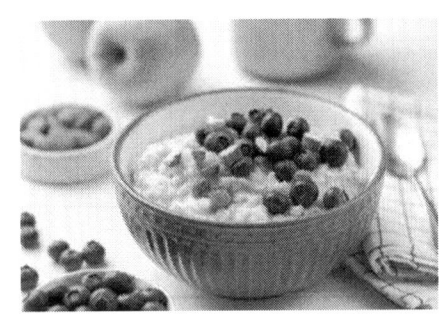

Nutritional Information per Serving

Calories: 269 calories
Fat: 3.6g
Sat. Fat: 0.4g
Carbohydrates: 49.3g
Protein: 11.7g
Fiber: 4.4g

Prep Time: 10 minutes | Cook Time: 20 minutes | Servings: 4; 1 bowl per serving

Ingredients

- 1 cup blueberries, fresh
- ½ of a lemon, zested
- 1 cups quinoa, rinsed
- 1/8 teaspoon salt
- ½ tablespoon and ½ teaspoon flax seeds
- 3 tablespoons honey, raw
- 2 cups almond milk, unsweetened, low-fat

Directions

- Take a medium saucepan, place it over medium heat, pour in the milk, and then cook for 3 minutes until thoroughly warmed.
- Add quinoa, stir in salt, switch heat to medium-low level and then cook for 20 minutes until the quinoa has absorbed all the milk.
- Then remove the pan from heat, stir in lemon zest and honey and then fold in berries until just mixed.
- Divide the quinoa evenly among four bowls and then serve.

Yogurt with Blueberries and Honey

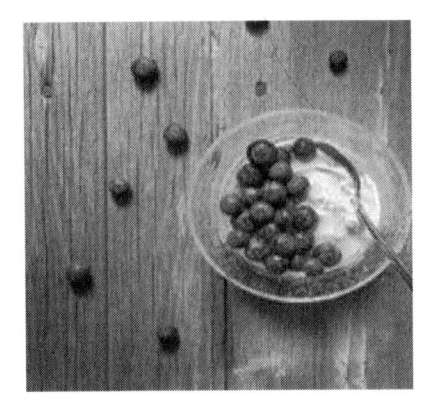

Nutritional Information per Serving

Calories: 196 calories
Fat: 1.1g
Sat. Fat: 0.3g
Carbohydrates: 24.6g
Protein: 23.5g
Fiber: 1.8g

Fat: 100 g

Prep Time: 10 minutes | Cook Time: 10 minutes | Servings: 4; 1 bowl per serving

Ingredients

- 2 cups blueberries, fresh
- 4 teaspoons honey
- 4 cups coconut yogurt or Greek yogurt, low-fat

Directions

- Take a small bowl, place 1 cup yogurt in it, top with ½ cup berries and then drizzle with 1 teaspoon honey.
- Assemble three more bowls in the same manner and then serve.

Chapter 7
Lunch

Tuna Patties

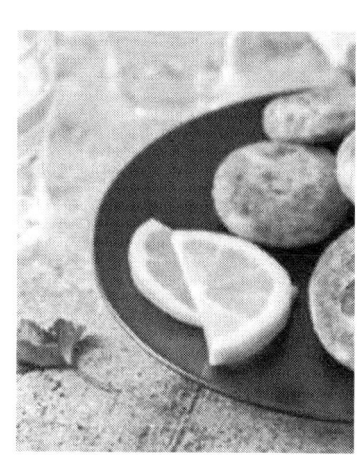

Nutritional Information per Serving

Calories: 216 calories
Fat: 12g
Sat. Fat: 3g
Carbohydrates: 32g
Protein: 12g
Fiber: 2g

Prep Time: 10 minutes | Cook Time: 15 minutes | Servings: 4; 2 patties per serving

Ingredients

- 14 ounces canned tuna, water-packed, drained
- 2 shallots, peeled, chopped
- 6 tablespoons bread crumbs
- 2 tablespoons parsley, chopped
- 4 tablespoons chives, chopped
- 2 tablespoons scallions,
- 2 tablespoons scallions, chopped
- ½ teaspoon ground black pepper
- 8 tablespoons whole-wheat flour
- 2/3 teaspoon salt

- chopped
- ½ teaspoon ground black pepper
- 4 tablespoons grated parmesan cheese
- 2 medium eggs, at room temperature
- 2 tablespoons sour cream
- 2 tablespoons olive oil

Directions

- Take a medium bowl, place tuna in it, add chopped shallots, bread crumbs, parsley, chives, scallion, black pepper, 4 tablespoons flour, salt, cheese, egg, and sour cream.
- Stir until well combined, shape the mixture into 8 evenly sized patties and then dredge in the remaining flour.
- Take a medium skillet pan, add oil and when hot, add prepared patties and then cook for 5 to 7 minutes per side until golden brown.
- Serve the tuna patties with a green salad.

Mediterranean Salmon

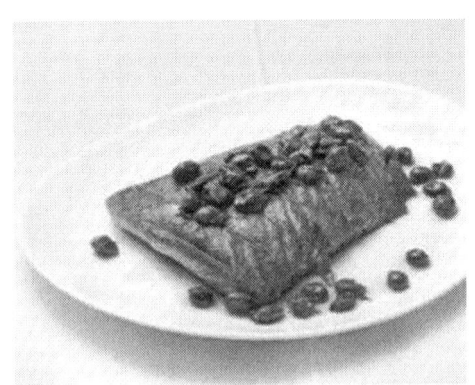

Nutritional Information per Serving

Calories: 301 calories
Fat: 15g
Sat. Fat: 2g
Carbohydrates: 5g
Protein: 35g
Fiber: 2g

Prep Time: 10 minutes | Cook Time: 25 minutes | Servings: 4; 1 piece per serving

Ingredients

- 1 ½ pound salmon fillet
- 1 tablespoon chopped dill
- ¼ teaspoon salt
- 2 teaspoons minced garlic
- 1/3 cup whole-grain mustard
- 1 tablespoon capers
- 2 tablespoons lemon juice
- 1 tablespoon olive oil
- 1 lemon, sliced

Directions

- Switch on the oven, then set it to 400 degrees F and let it preheat.
- Meanwhile, take a baking sheet and then place salmon fillet skin-side-down on it.
- Take a small bowl, place garlic, capers, dill, salt, and mustard in it, pour in the lemon juice and oil, and then stir until mixed.
- Brush the garlic mixture generously on the salmon, top with lemon slices, and then bake for 20 to 25 minutes until tender.
- Cut the salmon into four pieces and then serve.

Shrimp Linguine

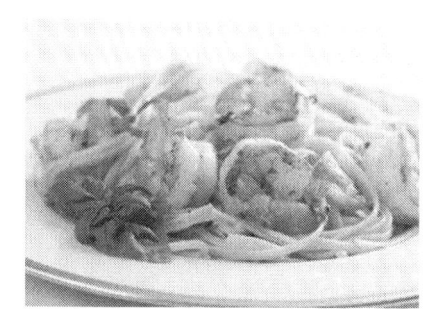

Nutritional Information per Serving

Calories: 231 calories
Fat: 8g
Sat. Fat: 1.5g
Carbohydrates: 24g
Protein: 1.5g
Fiber: 14g

Prep Time: 10 minutes | Cook Time: 25 minutes | Servings: 4; 1 plate per serving

Ingredients

- 12 ounces whole-wheat linguine
- 1 ½ pound medium shrimp, peeled, deveined
- ½ of a large white onion, peeled, chopped
- 1 teaspoon minced garlic
- 2/3 cup chopped roasted sweet red peppers
- 2-1/4 ounces sliced olives
- 1/3 cup minced parsley
- ½ teaspoon crushed red pepper flakes
- ½ teaspoon salt
- 2 tablespoons lemon juice
- ¼ teaspoon dried oregano
- ½ teaspoon ground black pepper
- 5 tablespoons olive oil
- 8 tablespoons crumbled feta cheese
- 1/3 cup chicken broth

Directions

- Prepare the pasta, and for this, take a large pot half full with water, place it over medium-high heat and then bring it to a boil.
- Add the pasta, cook it for 8 to 10 minutes until tender, then drain it well and reserve ½ cup of a cooking liquid, set aside until required.
- While pasta cooks, take a large skillet pan, place it over medium heat, add oil and when hot, add onion and cook for 2 to 3 minutes until onions begin to soften.
- Add shrimps, stir until just mixed, cook for 3 to 4 minutes per side until pink, stir in garlic and continue cooking for 1 minute.
- Switch heat to medium-low level, add olives, sweet red peppers, salt, parsley, black pepper, and oregano, pour in the reserved cooking liquid and stir until mixed.
- Add the cooked pasta along with cheese, drizzle with the lemon juice, stir until well mixed, cook for 3 to 4 minutes until the cheese has melted, and then serve.

Vegetarian Pasta Carbonara

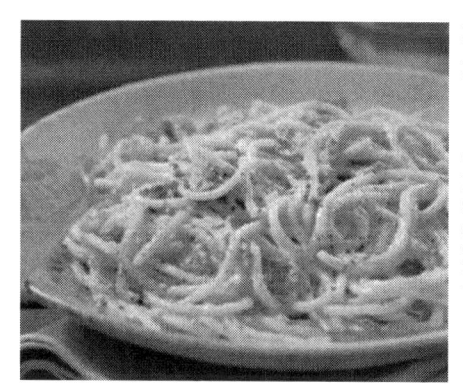

Nutritional Information per Serving

Calories: 300 calories
Fat: 11.5g
Sat. Fat: 3.5g
Carbohydrates: 36.5g
Protein: 12.5g
Fiber: 2.5g

Prep Time: 10 minutes | Cook Time: 22 minutes | Servings: 4; 1 bowl per serving

Ingredients

- 6 ounces whole-wheat spaghetti
- 1 tablespoon pine nuts, toasted
- 8 cherry tomatoes, halved
- 2 small zucchinis, cut into 1/3-inch-thick sticks
- ¼ teaspoon salt
- 1 teaspoon minced garlic
- 1/8 teaspoon ground black pepper
- 2 egg yolks, at room temperature
- 1 tablespoon olive oil and more as needed
- ½ cup grated parmesan, low-fat
- 3 tablespoons pasta water

Directions

- Take a large pot half full with salted water, place it over medium-high heat and then bring it to a boil.
- Add pasta, cook it for 10 to 12 minutes until tender, and then drain it into a colander, reserving 3 tablespoons of the pasta water.

- While pasta cooks, take a large frying pan, place it over medium heat, add oil and when hot, add zucchini and then cook for 5 to 8 minutes until nicely browned.
- Stir in garlic, cook for 1 minute, add tomatoes, stir in 1/8 teaspoon salt and then remove the pan from heat.
- Prepare the sauce and for this, take a medium bowl, place egg yolks in it, add cheese, black pepper, and remaining salt, whisk until smooth, and then whisk in the reserved pasta water until creamy sauce comes together.
- When zucchini has cooked, add the drained pasta, toss until combined, and then cook for 1 minute until thoroughly warmed.
- Pour in the prepared sauce, toss until mixed, sprinkle pine nuts and some more black pepper on top.
- Divide the pasta carbonara evenly among four plates and then serve.

Bean Burgers

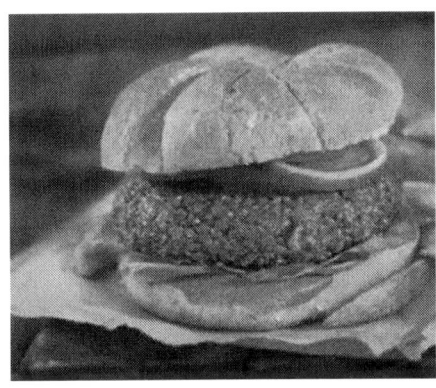

Nutritional Information per Serving

Calories: 323.3 calories
Fat: 23.3g
Sat. Fat: 4.4g
Carbohydrates: 16.6g
Protein: 11.1g
Fiber: 4g

Prep Time: 10 minutes | Cook Time: 15 minutes | Servings: 4 burgers; 1 burger per serving

Ingredients

For the Bean Patties:

- 24 ounces canned pink beans, rinsed
- ½ of a medium white onion, minced
- ½ cup chickpea flour
- 1/3 teaspoon ground black pepper
- 1 teaspoon minced garlic
- 1/3 teaspoon dried sage
- ¾ teaspoon salt
- ¾ teaspoon dried oregano
- ¾ cup chopped parsley
- ¼ cup olive oil
- 2 medium eggs, at room temperature

For the Burgers:

- 4 whole-wheat burger buns, halved, toasted
- 4 leaves of lettuce
- 4 slices of tomato
- 1 medium avocado, peeled, pitted, diced

Directions

- Prepare the bean patties, and for this, take a large bowl, place beans and onion in it and then add chickpea flour, black pepper, garlic, sage, salt, oregano, parsley, and eggs.
- Stir until well combined, and then shape the mixture into four evenly sized patties.
- Take a medium skillet pan, place it over medium-high heat, pour in the oil, and when hot, add the prepared bean patties and then cook for 6 to 8 minutes per side until golden brown.
- Assemble the burgers and for this, cut each burger bun in half and then toast the slices.
- Layer the bottom half of a burger bun with a lettuce leaf, and then place a bean patty on it.
- Top the bean patty with a tomato slice and avocado, drizzle with favorite sauce from the 'Sauces, Dips, and Dressing' section, and then cover with the top half of the bun.
- Assemble the remaining burgers in the same manner and then serve.

Herby Black Bean Salad with Feta Cheese

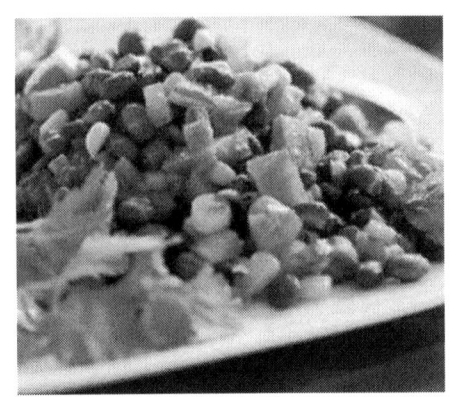

Nutritional Information per Serving

Calories: 245 calories
Fat: 15g
Sat. Fat: 3g
Carbohydrates: 23g
Protein: 9g
Fiber: 8g

Prep Time: 10 minutes | Cook Time: 0 minutes | Servings: 4; 1 bowl per serving

Ingredients

- 1 cup canned black beans, rinsed
- 2 roasted green peppers, chopped
- 2 cups arugula
- 2 scallions, chopped
- ¼ cup olives pitted
- ½ cup parsley leaves
- ½ teaspoon minced garlic
- ¼ teaspoon salt
- 2 cups diced tomatoes
- ¼ cup basil leaves
- 2 tablespoons pickled jalapenos
- ¼ teaspoon ground black pepper
- 4 tablespoons crumbled feta cheese, low-fat
- 2 tablespoons olive oil
- 2 tablespoons sesame seeds, toasted

Directions

- Take a medium bowl, place black beans and roasted green peppers along with arugula, scallion, olives, and tomatoes.
- Add remaining ingredients, toss until well combined, then divide the salad evenly among four bowls and serve.

Tomato, Basil, and Chickpea Salad

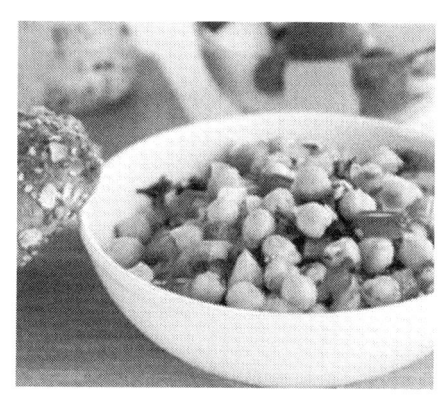

Nutritional Information per Serving

Calories: 354 calories
Fat: 18g
Sat. Fat: 3g
Carbohydrates: 35g
Protein: 13g
Fiber: 7g

Prep Time: 10 minutes | Cook Time: 10 minutes | Servings: 4; 1 bowl per serving

Ingredients

- 16 ounces canned chickpeas, drained, rinsed
- 3 small white onions, peeled, sliced
- 6 green onions, sliced
- 3 small red pepper, chopped
- 1 teaspoon salt
- 2 cups chopped cilantro
- 3 large tomatoes, chopped
- 1 cup basil leaves, chopped
- 4 tablespoons olive oil
- 4 tablespoons sesame seeds
- 4 teaspoons balsamic vinegar

Directions

- Take a large bowl, place chickpeas in it, and then add white onion, green onions, red pepper, and tomatoes.
- Season with salt, add cilantro and basil, drizzle with balsamic vinegar and then toss until just mixed.
- Sprinkle sesame seeds over the salad and then serve.

Tabouli Salad

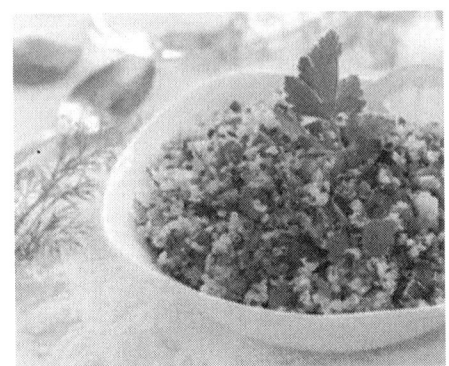

Nutritional Information per Serving

Calories: 257 calories
Fat: 13.3g
Sat. Fat: 4g
Carbohydrates: 34g
Protein: 4.3g
Fiber: 4.1g

Prep Time: 40 minutes | Cook Time: 0 minutes | Servings: 4; 1 bowl per serving

Ingredients

- ½ cup bulgur wheat
- 1 large cucumber, chopped
- 4 medium tomatoes, chopped
- 2 bunches of parsley, destemmed, chopped
- 4 green onions, green and white part separated, chopped
- 1 cup mint leaves, chopped
- ½ teaspoon salt

- 4 tablespoons lemon juice
- 3 tablespoons olive oil

Directions

- Wash the bulgur wheat, place it in a medium bowl, cover with water and then let the wheat soak for 5 to 7 minutes.
- Meanwhile, chop the tomatoes, place them into a colander and let them rest until excess juice has drained completely.
- Then take a large bowl, place tomatoes in it, and then add cucumber, green onion, parsley, and mint leaves.
- Add bulgur, season with salt, drizzle with lemon juice and olive oil, toss just mixed, and then cover the bowl with its lid.
- Place the bowl in the refrigerator, let it rest for 30 minutes, and then divide it evenly among four bowls.
- Serve the salad with Baba Ghanoush or hummus which you can prepare from the 'Sauces, Dips, and Dressing' section.

Roasted Eggplants

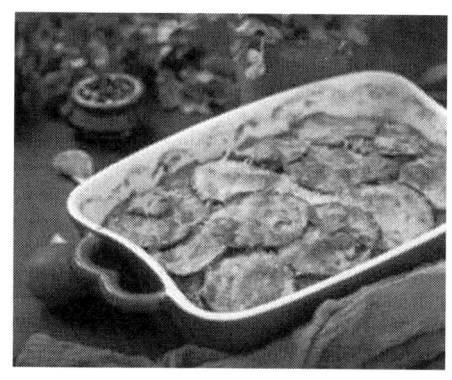

Nutritional Information per Serving

Calories: 249.7 calories
Fat: 17.2g
Sat. Fat: 4g
Carbohydrates: 18.7g
Protein: 5g
Fiber: 9g

Prep Time: 15 minutes | Cook Time: 1 hour and 10 minutes | Servings: 4

Ingredients

- 2 large eggplants, about 2-pounds total
- 4 medium tomatoes, chopped
- 5 cloves of garlic, peeled, minced
- 1 teaspoon salt
- ¼ cup chopped parsley
- ½ teaspoon ground black pepper
- ¼ cup chopped mint
- ¼ cup olive oil
- 3 tablespoons apple cider vinegar
- 4 tablespoons crumbled feta cheese, low-fat

Directions

- Cut the eggplant into ½-inch thick slices, place them in a large bowl, season with ½ teaspoon salt and then toss until just mixed.
- Take a large skillet pan, place it over medium-high heat, add 2 tablespoons of oil and when hot, spread eggplant slices in a single layer and then cook for 3 minutes per side until golden brown.
- Transfer the browned eggplant slices to a plate lined with a paper towel and then repeat with the remaining eggplant slices.
- Meanwhile, switch on the oven, set it to 350 degrees F, and let it preheat.
- When eggplant slices have cooked, return the skillet pan over medium heat, add garlic and cook for 1 to 2 minutes until fragrant and softened.
- Add tomatoes, season with black pepper and remaining salt, add vinegar and honey and then cook for 15 minutes or until thicken sauce comes together.
- Remove the pan from the heat, take a medium baking dish, spread a few tablespoons of the sauce in its bottom, and then drizzle with a little oil.
- Layer with eggplant slices in a single layer and sprinkle with some parsley, mint, and feta cheese.
- Spread some of the prepared tomato sauce over the eggplant layer and then continue layering remaining eggplant slices with parsley, mint, feta cheese, and tomato sauce until all of these ingredients have used up.
- Use a spatula to press down the eggplant slices, drizzle vinegar on top and then bake for 45 minutes until done.
- Sprinkle some more feta cheese on top and then serve.

Mediterranean Cauliflower Pizza

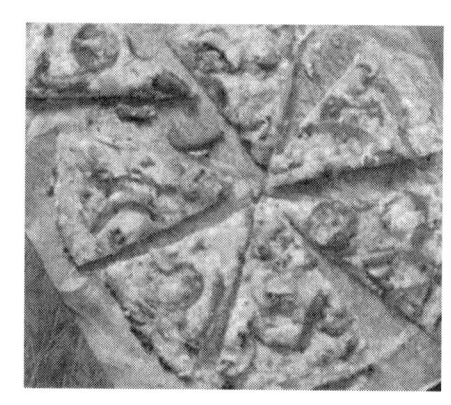

Nutritional Information per Serving

Calories: 200 calories
Fat: 14g
Sat. Fat: 4.7g
Carbohydrates: 10.2g
Protein: 10.8g
Fiber: 3.2g

Prep Time: 15 minutes | Cook Time: 35 minutes | Servings: 1 pizza; 1 slice per serving

Ingredients

- 2 pounds head of cauliflower, chopped into florets
- 6 sun-dried tomatoes, oil-packed, drained, chopped
- ½ teaspoon dried oregano
- ⅓ cup olives, pitted, sliced
- ½ teaspoon ground black pepper
- ¼ teaspoon salt
- 1 tablespoon and 1 teaspoon olive oil, divided
- 1 large lemon
- 1 large egg, at room temperature, beaten
- ¼ cup sliced basil
- 1 cup shredded mozzarella cheese, low-fat

Directions

- Switch on the oven, then set it to 450 degrees F and let it preheat.
- Meanwhile, take a pizza pan, line it with parchment paper, and set it aside until required.
- Plug in a food processor, place cauliflower florets in it, and then pulse until mixture resembles rice.
- Take a large skillet pan, place it over medium heat, add 1 tablespoon oil and when hot, add cauliflower mixture, stir in salt and then cook for 8 to 10 minutes until golden brown.
- Then transfer the cauliflower mixture into a large bowl and then let it cool at room temperature for 10 minutes.
- Meanwhile, peel the lemon, remove and discard its white pith, remove the seeds, and then cut the lemon into segments.
- Drain the juice from the lemon segment, place the lemon pieces into a bowl, add olives and tomatoes and then toss until combined.
- When the cauliflower mixture has cooled, add cheese, oregano, and egg, stir until well combined, spoon the mixture into the prepared pizza pan, and then spread it evenly.
- Drizzle the remaining oil on top, place it into the oven, and then bake for 10 to 15 minutes until the crust begins to turn brown.
- Then scatter the prepared olives-tomato-lemon mixture over the top of the baked crust, season with the black pepper, and continue baking the pizza for 8 to 14 minutes until done.
- Scatter basil leaves on top, cut into slices and then serve.

Quinoa and Avocado Salad

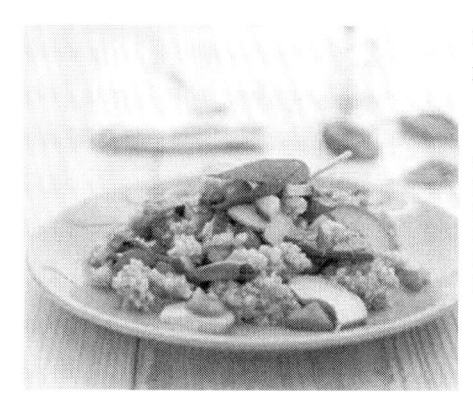

Nutritional Information per Serving

Calories: 236 calories
Fat: 5.7g
Sat. Fat: 1.8g
Carbohydrates: 25.2g
Protein: 5.2g
Fiber: 6.7g

Prep Time: 25 minutes | Cook Time: 15 minutes | Servings: 4; 1 bowl per serving

Ingredients

For the Salad Dressing:

- ¾ teaspoon salt
- ¾ teaspoon garlic powder
- ¼ teaspoon ground black pepper
- 2 tablespoons avocado oil
- 3 tablespoons lime juice

For the Salad:

- 1 medium avocado, peeled, pitted, chopped
- ¾ cup quinoa, uncooked, rinsed
- ½ cup grape tomatoes, halved
- ½ cup spinach leaves, fresh
- 1 scallion, sliced
- ¾ cup diced cucumber
- ¼ cup chopped cilantro
- 1 ½ cup water

Directions

- Prepare the quinoa, and for this, take a medium pot, pour water in it, place it over medium-high heat and bring it to a boil.
- Then switch heat to medium level, add quinoa and then cook for 8 to 15 minutes until all the liquid has been absorbed by the quinoa.
- Meanwhile, prepare the salad dressing and for this, take a small bowl, place all the ingredients for the dressing in it and then stir until combined, set aside until required.
- Remove the pot from heat, cover it with its lid, let the quinoa rest for 5 minutes, and then fluff it with a fork.
- Stir ¼ teaspoon salt into the quinoa, and then let the quinoa rest for 15 minutes at room temperature.
- Take a large bowl, place quinoa in it, add the remaining ingredients of the salad in it, drizzle with the prepared salad dressing, and then stir gently until just mixed.
- Divide the salad between 4 bowls and then serve.

Chickpea and Quinoa Bowl

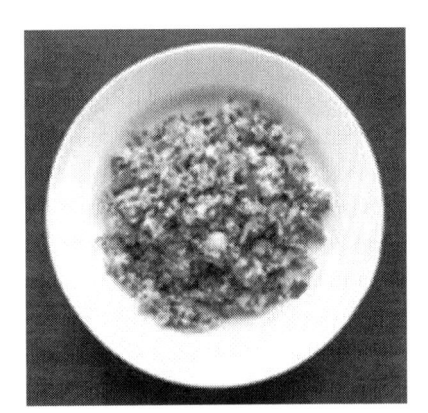

Nutritional Information per Serving

Calories: 273 calories
Fat: 24.3g
Sat. Fat: 4.3g
Carbohydrates: 49g
Protein: 12.7g
Fiber: 7.7g

Prep Time: 25 minutes | Cook Time: 15 minutes | Servings: 4; 1 bowl per serving

Ingredients

For the Salad Dressing:

- 7 ounces roasted red peppers, rinsed
- ¼ cup slivered almonds
- 2 tablespoons olive oil
- ¼ teaspoon crushed red pepper
- ½ teaspoon ground cumin
- ½ teaspoon minced garlic

For the Salad:

- ½ cup quinoa, uncooked, rinsed
- ¼ cup Kalamata olives, chopped
- 12 ounces canned chickpeas, drained, rinsed
- ¼ cup chopped red onion
- ½ cup diced cucumber
- ½ teaspoon paprika
- 1 ½ tablespoon olive oil
- ¼ cup crumbled feta cheese, low-fat
- 2 tablespoons chopped parsley
- 1 cup water

Directions

- Prepare the quinoa, and for this, take a medium pot, pour water in it, place it over medium-high heat and bring it to a boil.
- Then switch heat to medium level, add quinoa and then cook for 8 to 15 minutes until all the liquid has been absorbed by the quinoa.
- Meanwhile, prepare the salad dressing and for this, plug in a food processor, add all the ingredients for the salad dressing in it and then pulse until smooth.
- Remove the pot from heat, cover it with its lid, let the quinoa rest for 5 minutes, and then fluff it with a fork.
- Stir ¼ teaspoon salt into the quinoa, and then let the quinoa rest for 15 minutes at room temperature.
- Take a large bowl, place quinoa in it, add the remaining ingredients of the salad in it, drizzle with the prepared salad dressing, and then stir gently until just mixed.
- Divide the salad between 4 bowls and then serve.

Chapter 8

Snacks

Pineapple and Green Smoothie

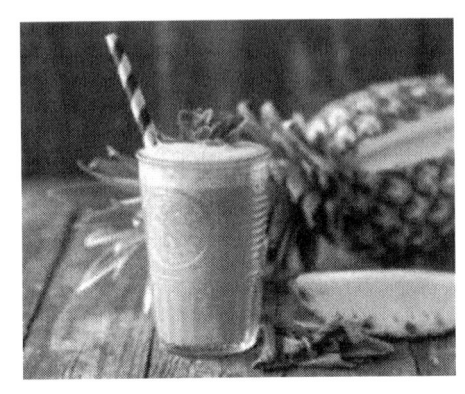

Nutritional Information per Serving

Calories: 195 calories
Fat: 3g
Sat. Fat: 1.1g
Carbohydrates: 32.6g
Protein: 9.3g
Fiber: 5.1g

Prep Time: 5 minutes | Cook Time: 0 minutes | Servings: 1 glass

Ingredients

- ¼ cup almond milk, unsweetened
- ¼ cup Greek yogurt, low-fat
- ½ cup baby spinach, fresh
- ¼ cup pineapple chunks, frozen
- 1 frozen banana, peeled
- 1 Medjool date, pitted
- 1 teaspoon chia seeds

Directions

- Plugin the food processor and then pour milk and yogurt in its jar.
- Add spinach, pineapple, banana, honey, and chia seeds, and then pulse for 30 seconds or more until smooth.
- Pour the smoothie into a glass and then serve.

Tahini and Date Shake

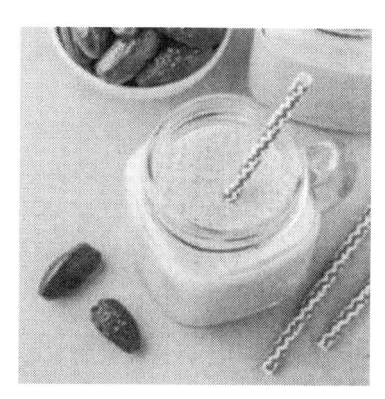

Nutritional Information per Serving

Calories: 199.4 calories
Fat: 8.2g
Sat. Fat: 1.6g
Carbohydrates: 27.7g
Protein: 3.7g
Fiber: 5.6g

Prep Time: 5 minutes | Cook Time: 0 minutes | Servings: 1

Ingredients

- ¼ cup ice cubes
- ½ cup almond milk, unsweetened
- 1 frozen banana, peeled
- 1 ½ tablespoon tahini
- 1 Medjool date, pitted
- ¼ teaspoon ground cinnamon

Directions

- Plugin the food processor, add ice cubes, and then pour in the milk.
- Add banana, tahini, date, and cinnamon, and then pulse for 30 seconds or more until smooth.
- Pour the smoothie into a glass and then serve.

Chia and Pomegranate Smoothie

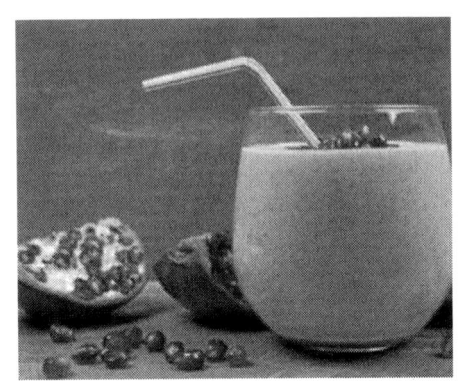

Nutritional Information per Serving

Calories: 208 calories
Fat: 4.6g
Sat. Fat: 1.3g
Carbohydrates: 32.7g
Protein: 8.8g
Fiber: 4.9g

Prep Time: 5 minutes | Cook Time: 0 minutes | Servings: 1

Ingredients

- ½ cup pomegranate juice, chilled
- ¼ cup Greek yogurt, low-fat
- ½ of a frozen banana, peeled
- 1 tablespoon chia seeds

Directions

- Plugin the food processor and then pour in the juice and yogurt.
- Add banana and chia seeds, and then pulse for 30 seconds or more until smooth.
- Pour the smoothie into a glass and then serve.

Orange Salad

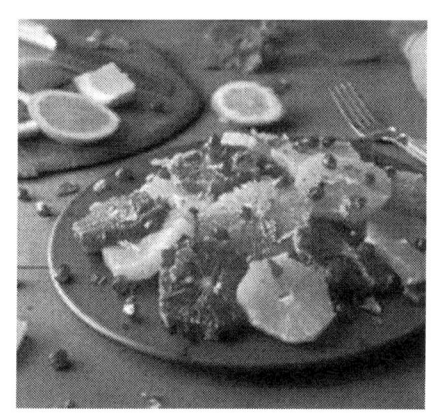

Nutritional Information per Serving

Calories: 186 calories
Fat: 11.7g
Sat. Fat: 1.6g
Carbohydrates: 21.4g
Protein: 1.8g
Fiber: 4.5g

Prep Time: 5 minutes | Cook Time: 0 minutes | Servings: 4; 1 plate per serving

Ingredients

- 4 oranges
- 1 small white onion, peeled, diced
- 3 blood oranges
- 1/8 teaspoon salt
- 2 tablespoons lemon juice
- 1/8 teaspoon ground black pepper
- 10 dried black olives
- 3 tablespoons olive oil

Directions

- Prepare the oranges and for this, cut off a small piece from its top and bottom, remove the skin and white pith, and then cut the oranges into horizontal slices.
- Take a small bowl, place onion slices in it, add salt, lemon juice, and olive oil and then stir until combined.
- Spoon the onion mixture over the orange slices, season with black pepper, and then scatter olives from the top.
- Serve straight away.

Mediterranean Fruit Salad

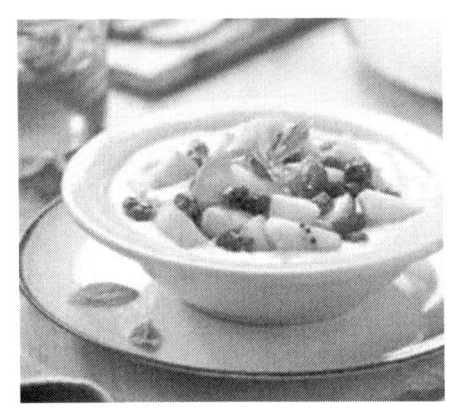

Nutritional Information per Serving

Calories: 201 calories
Fat: 0.9g
Sat. Fat: 0.1g
Carbohydrates: 51.3g
Protein: 2.6g
Fiber: 9.1g

Prep Time: 5 minutes | Cook Time: 0 minutes | Servings: 4; 1 bowl per serving

Ingredients

- 2 medium pears, cored, chopped
- 24 grapes, seedless
- 2 medium apples, cored, chopped
- 2 medium peaches, chopped
- 2 oranges, peeled, deseeded, chopped

- 4 kiwi fruits, chopped
- 1 cup Greek yogurt, low-fat

Directions

- Take a large bowl and then place pears, grapes, apples, kiwi, peaches, and oranges.
- Add yogurt, stir until well mixed and then divide the salad evenly among four bowls.
- Serve straight away.

Trail Mix

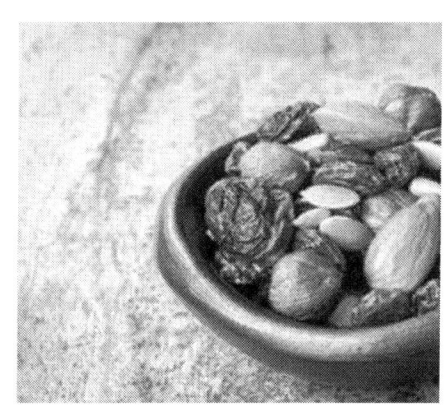

Nutritional Information per Serving

Calories: 218.5 calories
Fat: 12.4g
Sat. Fat: 2.3g
Carbohydrates: 21.3g
Protein: 5.5g
Fiber: 5.5g

Prep Time: 10 minutes | Cook Time: 0 minutes | Servings: 4; 1 bowl per serving

Ingredients

For the Trail Mix:
- 2 tablespoons whole dried cherries
- 12 apricots, dried

- 2 tablespoons sunflower seeds, unsalted
- ½ cup almonds
- 3 tablespoons chocolate chips, semi-sweetened

For Each Serving:

- ½ cup almond milk, unsweetened, low-fat

Directions

- Take a large bowl, place sunflower seeds, almonds, chocolate chips, cherries, and apricot, and then stir until mixed.
- Transfer the prepared trail mix into a resealable glass container and then store it at room temperature until required.
- When ready to serve, transfer ½ cup of the trail mix into a bowl, pour in ½ cup milk, and then serve.

Flatbread Crackers

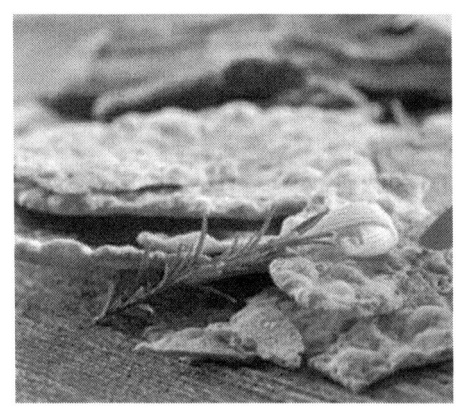

Nutritional Information per Serving

Calories: 190 calories
Fat: 6g
Sat. Fat: 1g
Carbohydrates: 29g
Protein: 4g
Fiber: 1.2g

Prep Time: 10 minutes | Cook Time: 10 minutes | Servings: 4

Ingredients

- 1 ½ cups whole-wheat flour
- 1 teaspoon ground black pepper
- 2 teaspoons dried thyme
- 1 teaspoon coconut sugar
- 1 teaspoon salt
- 2 tablespoons olive oil
- ½ cup water, chilled

Directions

- Switch on the oven, then set it to 450 degrees F and let it preheat.
- Meanwhile, plug in a food processor, add flour in it, add salt, sugar, black pepper, and thyme, and then pour in olive oil.
- Pulse until well mixed, and then slowly blend in water for 10 seconds until a sticky dough comes together.

- Transfer the dough to a clean working space dusted with flour, shape it into a ball, divide the ball into four evenly sized portions, and then let the dough portions rest for 10 minutes.
- Meanwhile, take a baking sheet, line it with a parchment sheet, and set it aside until required.
- Working on one portion of dough at a time, roll it as thin as possible, transfer it to the prepared baking sheet and bake for 4 to 5 minutes per side until golden brown.
- When done, switch off the oven and then let the cracker rest in the oven for 1 to 2 hours until dried and crisp.
- Then break the crispy cracker into pieces and repeat with the remaining flour portions.
- Serve the crackers with your favorite dip, which you can prepare from the 'Sauces, Dips, and Dressing' section.

Roasted Chickpeas

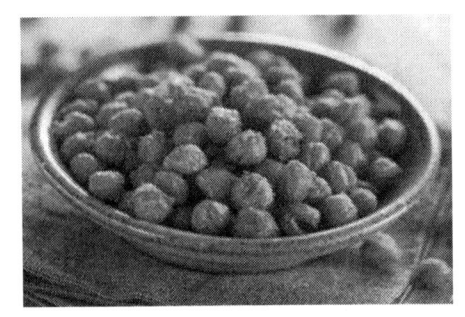

Nutritional Information per Serving

Calories: 208 calories
Fat: 9.4g
Sat. Fat: 1.1g
Carbohydrates: 23.8g
Protein: 6.7g
Fiber: 6.8g

Prep Time: 10 minutes | Cook Time: 30 minutes | Servings: 4

Ingredients

- 15 ounces canned chickpeas, drained, rinsed
- ¼ teaspoon garlic powder
- ½ teaspoon salt
- 2 tablespoons olive oil
- 1 teaspoon dried oregano
- 2 teaspoons red wine vinegar
- ¼ teaspoon ground black pepper
- 2 teaspoons lemon juice

Directions

- Switch on the oven, then set it to 425 degrees F and let it preheat.
- Meanwhile, take a large baking sheet and then line it with the parchment.
- Spread the chickpeas into the prepared baking sheet in a single layer and then roast for 20 minutes until golden brown, stirring halfway.
- Meanwhile, prepare the dressing and for this, take a large bowl, place garlic powder, salt, black pepper, and oregano in it, pour in lemon juice and olive oil, and then whisk until well combined.

- When the chickpeas have roasted, transfer them into the bowl containing prepared dressing and then toss until coated.
- Spoon the chickpeas into the baking sheet, spread them in a single layer, and then roast them for 10 minutes, stirring halfway.
- Let the roasted chickpeas cool for 5 minutes and then serve.

Baked Zucchini Sticks

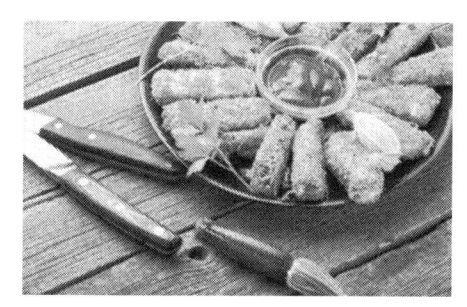

Nutritional Information per Serving

Calories: 132 calories
Fat: 6.6g
Sat. Fat: 3.6g
Carbohydrates: 9.6g
Protein: 10.8g
Fiber: 3.2g

Prep Time: 10 minutes | Cook Time: 25 minutes | Servings: 4

Ingredients

- 4 large zucchinis, ends trimmed, cut into lengthwise sticks
- 6 tablespoons olive oil

For the Topping:

- ¾ teaspoon salt
- 3 teaspoons dried thyme
- 1 teaspoon paprika
- 2 teaspoons dried oregano
- 1 teaspoon ground black pepper
- 1 cup grated parmesan cheese, low-fat

Directions

- Switch on the oven, then set it to 350 degrees F and let it preheat.
- Meanwhile, take a shallow dish, place all the ingredients for the topping in it and then stir until just mixed.
- Take a large baking sheet, place a wire rack on it, and then brush it with oil.
- Arrange the prepared zucchini sticks skin-side-down on the wire rack in a single layer, brush them with oil and then sprinkle with the prepared topping mixture until coated.
- Place the prepared baking tray into the oven to bake for 20 minutes until golden crisp, then switch on the broiler and continue baking the zucchini sticks for 3 minutes.
- When done, serve the zucchini sticks with your favorite sauce, which you can prepare from the '<u>Sauces, Dips, and Dressing</u>' section.

Fish Sticks

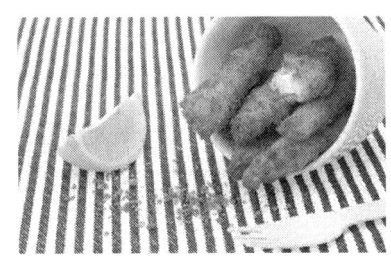

Nutritional Information per Serving

Calories: 238 calories
Fat: 7.6g
Sat. Fat: 2.2g
Carbohydrates: 16g
Protein: 27.2g
Fiber: 1.2g

Prep Time: 15 minutes | Cook Time: 18 minutes | Servings: 16 fish sticks; 4 fish sticks per serving

Ingredients

- ½ cup whole-wheat breadcrumbs
- 1½ pounds cod, skinless
- ½ cup whole-wheat flour
- 1 teaspoon salt
- 1 teaspoon dried oregano
- 1 teaspoon ground black pepper
- 1 teaspoon sweet paprika
- 1 lemon, zested
- 1 large egg, at room temperature
- ½ cup grated Parmesan cheese, low-fat
- ½ of a lemon, juiced
- 4 tablespoons olive oil
- 1 tablespoon chopped parsley

Directions

- Switch on the oven, then set it to 450 degrees F and let it preheat.
- Rinse the fish, pat dry with paper towels, season well with salt, and then cut it into 3-inch-long slices, each about 1 ½ inch thick.
- Take a small bowl, place paprika, oregano, and black pepper in it, stir until well mixed and then sprinkle this mixture on the fish sticks until coated.
- Take a shallow dish and then place flour in it.
- Take another shallow dish, crack the egg in it and then whisk until blended.
- Take another shallow dish, place breadcrumbs in it, add lemon zest and parmesan cheese, and then stir until mixed.
- Working on one fish stick at a time, dredge it in flour, dip into the blended eggs and then dredge in the breadcrumbs mixture until well coated.
- Take a large baking sheet, grease it with oil, arrange the prepared fish sticks on it, brush some more oil on top of the prepared fish sticks and then bake for 15 minutes until golden brown, turning halfway.
- Then switch on the broiler and continue baking the fish sticks for 3 minutes.
- When done, sprinkle lemon zest over the fish sticks, drizzle with lemon juice and then sprinkle parsley over the top.
- Serve the fish sticks with your favorite sauce, which you can prepare from the 'Sauces, Dips, and Dressing' section.

Kale Chips

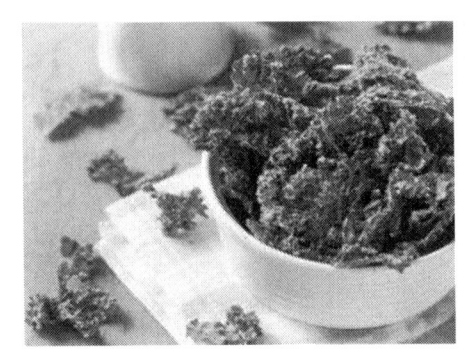

Nutritional Information per Serving

Calories: 176 calories
Fat: 16g
Sat. Fat: 3g
Carbohydrates: 4.4g
Protein: 3.4g
Fiber: 2.4g

Prep Time: 10 minutes | Cook Time: 30 minutes | Servings: 4

Ingredients

- 8 cups kale leaves
- 2 teaspoons lemon zest
- ½ teaspoon salt
- 2 teaspoons Italian seasoning
- ½ teaspoon ground black pepper
- 4 tablespoons olive oil
- 4 tablespoons grated parmesan cheese, low-fat

Directions

- Switch on the oven, then set it to 350 degrees F and let it preheat.
- Take a large baking sheet, line it with baking paper, and then spread the kale leaves in a single layer.
- Season kale leaves with salt, black pepper, lemon zest, and parmesan cheese, drizzle with oil, toss until mixed, and then massage the leaves for 2 minutes.
- Place the prepared baking sheet containing kale leaves into the oven and bake for 15 minutes until crisp, turning halfway.

- When done, let the kale leaves rest until crisp further and repeat with the remaining kale leaves.

Vegetable Chips

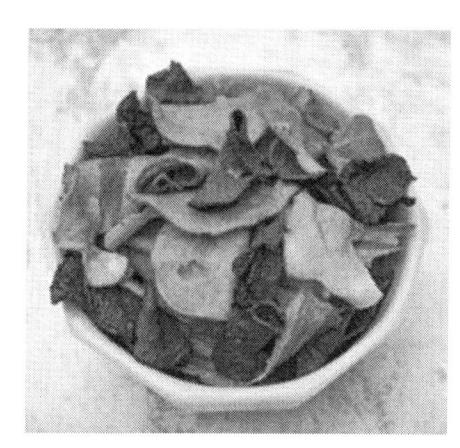

Nutritional Information per Serving

Calories: 100 calories
Fat: 5g
Sat. Fat: 1g
Carbohydrates: 14g
Protein: 2g
Fiber: 6g

Prep Time: 15 minutes | Cook Time: 30 minutes | Servings: 4

Ingredients

- 2 medium beetroots, peeled
- 1 medium rutabaga, peeled
- 1 large zucchini, peeled
- 1 small sweet potato, peeled
- 1 teaspoon salt
- 1 teaspoon garlic powder
- ½ teaspoon ground black pepper
- ½ cup olive oil

Directions

- Switch on the oven, then set it to 450 degrees F and let it preheat.
- Meanwhile, take 2 large rimmed baking sheets, line them with foil and then brush them with oil, set them aside until required.
- Peel the vegetables, cut them into 1/8-inch-thick slices, and then spread them in a single layer on the prepared baking sheets.
- Brush the top of vegetable slices with the remaining oil and then sprinkle with garlic powder, salt, and black pepper.
- Place the prepared baking sheets into the oven and then bake for 30 minutes until nicely browned and crisp, turning halfway.
- Serve the vegetable chips with your favorite dip, which you can prepare from the 'Sauces, Dips, and Dressing' section.

Chapter 9

Dinner

Cod with Tomatoes and Olives

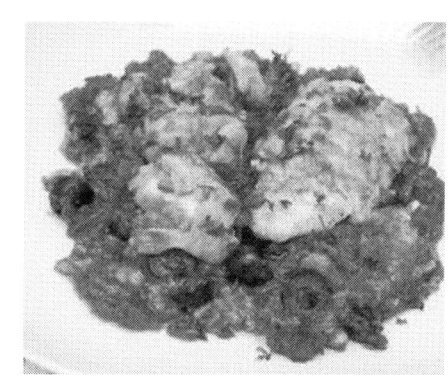

Nutritional Information per Serving

Calories: 256 calories
Fat: 16g
Sat. Fat: 3g
Carbohydrates: 6g
Protein: 24g
Fiber: 3g

Prep Time: 10 minutes | Cook Time: 15 minutes | Servings: 4; 1 plate per serving

Ingredients

- 1 pound fillet of cod, deboned
- ¼ cup basil leaves, chopped
- 10 ounces baby spinach, fresh
- 1 teaspoon salt
- 1/3 cup kalamata olives, sliced
- ½ teaspoon ground black pepper
- ¼ cup sun-dried tomatoes,
- ¼ cup parsley leaves, chopped
- 6 pepperoncini, sliced
- ½ teaspoon red pepper flakes
- 2 tablespoons olive oil
- ¼ cup pine nuts
- ¼ cup crumbled feta cheese, low-

| sliced, packed in oil | fat |

Directions

- Switch on the oven, then set it to 400 degrees F and let it preheat.
- Take a baking dish about the size of a fish fillet, grease it with 1 tablespoon oil, scatter spinach leaves in the bottom and then top with the fillet, skin-side-down.
- Sprinkle salt and black pepper over the fillet, drizzle with remaining, top with tomatoes, olives, nuts, and pepperoncini, and then sprinkle with the red pepper flakes.
- Sprinkle basil leaves and parsley leaves over the fillet, and bake the fish for 10 minutes.
- Then sprinkle feta cheese over the fish, continue baking for 5 minutes and then serve.

Grilled Sea Bass

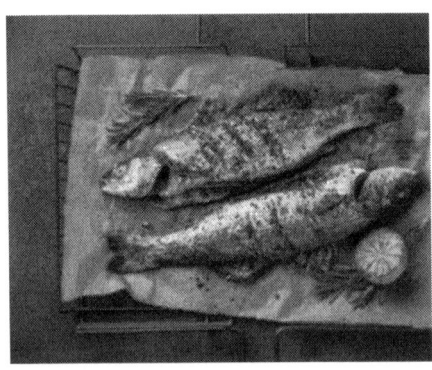

Nutritional Information per Serving

Calories: 305 calories
Fat: 15g
Sat. Fat: 3g
Carbohydrates: 1g
Protein: 40g
Fiber: 0g

Prep Time: 25 minutes | Cook Time: 20 minutes | Servings: 4

Ingredients

- 2 whole sea bass, about 1 ½ pounds, cleaned
- 1 ¼ teaspoon salt
- 2 tablespoons lemon juice
- 1 tablespoon chopped oregano leaves
- 1 tablespoon lemon zest
- ¼ teaspoon ground black pepper
- 3 tablespoons olive oil
- 1 teaspoon ground coriander
- 2 large sprigs of oregano
- 1 lemon, cut into wedges

Directions

- Take a small bowl, place lemon zest, coriander, oregano, and ¼ teaspoon salt, pour in lemon juice and oil, and then stir until mixed.
- Pat dry the sea bass with paper towels, make three cuts into each fish and then season with black pepper and remaining salt.
- Stuff each fish with oregano sprigs and lemon wedges and arrange them into a baking dish.
- Rub the fishes with half of the prepared oil mixture and let them rest for 15 minutes.
- Meanwhile, take a griddle pan, grease it with oil, place it over medium-high heat and let it preheat.
- Place the prepared fish on the griddle pan and then cook for 15 to 20 minutes until fork-tender, turning halfway.
- When done, transfer fish to a cutting board, make a cut along the backbone of the fish, use a spatula to lift out the backbone and ribs, and discard them.
- Repeat with the other fish, transfer fish to a plate, drizzle the remaining oil mixture on top and then serve.

Shrimp in Garlic Sauce

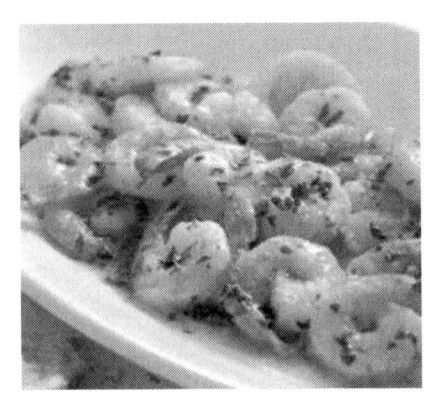

Nutritional Information per Serving

Calories: 268.5 calories
Fat: 12.1g
Sat. Fat: 1.6g
Carbohydrates: 1.8g
Protein: 37.5g
Fiber: 0.75g

Prep Time: 5 minutes | Cook Time: 10 minutes | Servings: 4

Ingredients

- 1 ½ pound shrimps, peeled, deveined
- 6 teaspoons minced garlic
- 1 ½ teaspoon salt
- 1 ½ tablespoon lemon juice
- ¾ teaspoon ground black pepper
- ½ teaspoon red pepper flakes
- 1/3 tablespoon vegetable broth
- 3 tablespoons olive oil

Directions

- Take a large skillet pan, place it over medium heat, add oil and when hot, add garlic and cook for 1 minute until fragrant.
- Add shrimps, season with salt, black pepper, and red pepper flakes, pour in the lemon juice, stir until mixed, and then cook for 1 minute.

- Then switch heat to the low level, pour in the broth, stir until just mixed, and then cook for 5 to 8 minutes until the shrimps turn pink.
- Serve shrimps alone or over the cooked whole-wheat pasta.

Greek Turkey Burgers

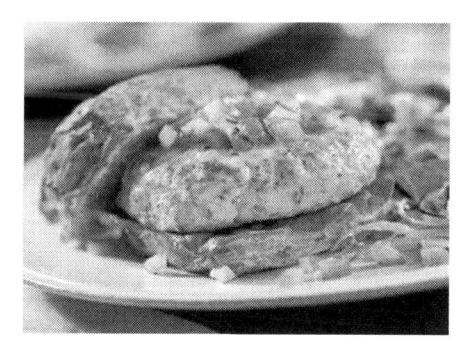

Nutritional Information per Serving

Calories: 376 calories
Fat: 17g
Sat. Fat: 6.2g
Carbohydrates: 28.5g
Protein: 30g
Fiber: 5g

Prep Time: 15 minutes | Cook Time: 10 minutes | Servings: 4; 1 burger per serving

Ingredients

- 1 cup chopped spinach, fresh or thawed if frozen
- 1 pound ground turkey, extra-lean
- ½ teaspoon garlic powder
- ¼ teaspoon salt
- ½ teaspoon dried oregano
- ¼ teaspoon ground black pepper
- 1 cup chopped spinach, fresh or thawed if frozen
- 1 pound ground turkey, extra-lean
- ½ teaspoon garlic powder
- ¼ teaspoon salt
- ½ teaspoon dried oregano
- ¼ teaspoon ground black pepper

Directions

- Squeeze the spinach to remove excess water and then place it in a large bowl.

- Add ground turkey, salt, black pepper, oregano, garlic powder, and feta cheese, stir until well combined, and then shape the mixture into four evenly sized patties.
- Take a griddle pan, grease it with oil, place it over medium-high heat and let it preheat.
- Arrange the prepared patties on the griddle pan and then cook for 5 to 8 minutes per side until golden brown and thoroughly cooked.
- Assemble the burgers and for this, take a bottom half of the hamburger, place a turkey patty on it and then spoon 1 tablespoon of the prepared tzatziki sauce on it.
- Top with 3 slices of cucumber, 2 onion rings, and then cover with the top half of the hamburger.
- Prepare the remaining burgers in the same manner and then serve.

Grilled Chicken Kabobs

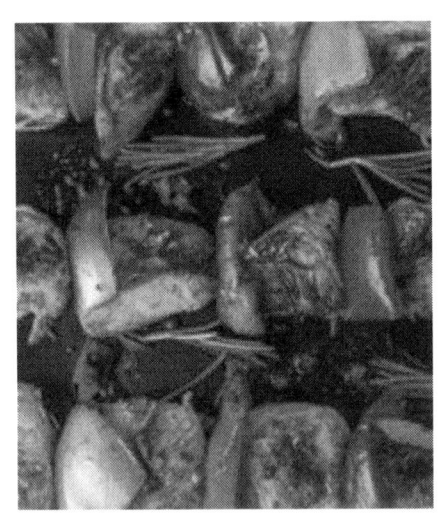

Nutritional Information per Serving

Calories: 296 calories
Fat: 20.4g
Sat. Fat: 3g
Carbohydrates: 12.2g
Protein: 17.6g
Fiber: 2.8g

Prep Time: 2 hours and 15 minutes | Cook Time: 20 minutes | Servings: 24 skewers; 6 skewers per serving

Ingredients

- 4 pounds chicken breasts, boneless, skinless, 1 ½-inch cubed
- 2 medium green bell peppers, cored, cut into 1 ½-inch piece
- 2 large white onions, peeled, sliced
- 2 medium red bell peppers, cored, cut into 1 ½-inch piece
- 2 teaspoons ground nutmeg
- 3 teaspoons salt
- ½ teaspoon ground cardamom
- 2 teaspoons dried thyme
- 2 teaspoons ground black pepper
- 3 teaspoons paprika
- 25 cloves of garlic, peeled, minced
- 1 cup olive oil
- 2 medium red onions, cored, cut into 1 ½-inch piece
- 5 lemons, juiced
- Tahini sauce as needed for serving (prepare from the 'Sauces, Dips, and Dressing' section)

Directions

- Prepare a spice mix and for this, take a small bowl, place ¼ teaspoon each of salt and black pepper along with thyme, cardamom, paprika, and nutmeg and then stir until mixed.
- Take a large bowl, place chicken pieces in it, add prepared spice mix, and then toss well until coated.
- Add white onion slices and garlic, drizzle with lemon juice and oil, toss until coated, cover the bowl with its lid, place it in the refrigerator and let it rest for 4 hours.
- When ready to cook, take a griddle pan, grease it with oil, place it over medium-high heat and let it preheat.
- Thread chicken pieces, red onion, and bell pepper slices onto wooden skewers, arrange the skewers on the griddle pan, and cook for 10 to 12 minutes or more until thoroughly cooked.
- Serve the chicken skewers with tahini sauce.

Sweet and Sour Chicken

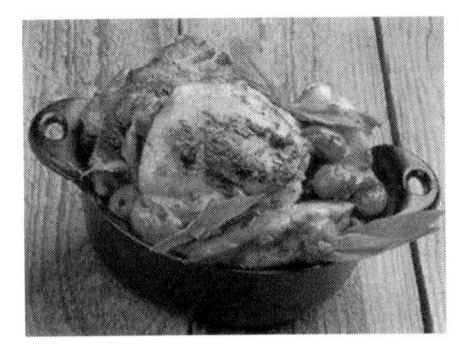

Nutritional Information per Serving

Calories: 375 calories
Fat: 11g
Sat. Fat: 2g
Carbohydrates: 30g
Protein: 38g
Fiber: 5g

Prep Time: 10 minutes | Cook Time: 35 minutes | Servings: 4; 1 plate per serving

Ingredients

- 2 pounds chicken thighs, boneless, skinless
- ¾ cup figs, halved
- 1 tablespoon minced garlic
- 2 teaspoons cornstarch
- ¼ teaspoon salt
- 2 teaspoons coconut sugar
- 2 teaspoons olive oil
- ¼ cup red wine vinegar
- ½ cup chicken broth
- ¼ cup salad olives, stuffed
- 5 ounces baby arugula, fresh

Directions

- Take a large skillet pan, place it over medium-high heat, add oil, and when hot, add chicken thighs.
- Season them with salt and then cook for 17 to 20 minutes until the chicken turns nicely golden brown and thoroughly cooked, covering the pan with its lid.
-

- When done, transfer the chicken thighs to a plate, add minced garlic into the skillet pan and then cook for 30 seconds until fragrant.
- Meanwhile, take a medium bowl, pour in the broth and vinegar, and then whisk in sugar and cornstarch until blended.
- Pour the broth mixture into the skillet pan, stir well to loosen browned bits at the bottom of the pan, and then bring the sauce to a boil.
- Continue boiling the sauce for 1 minute or more until thickened to the desired level, add olives, chicken thighs, and figs and then cook for 3 to 4 minutes until thoroughly hot.
- Divide the arugula among four plates, top with the chicken and its sauce, and then serve.

Hasselback Caprese Chicken

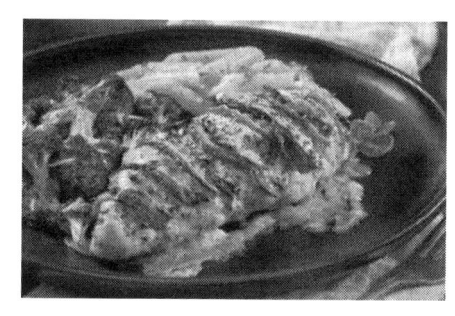

Nutritional Information per Serving

Calories: 311 calories
Fat: 15.9g
Sat. Fat: 5.9g
Carbohydrates: 9g
Protein: 32.6g
Fiber: 4.2g

Prep Time: 15 minutes | Cook Time: 25 minutes | Servings: 4

Ingredients

- 2 chicken breasts, skinless, boneless, each about 8 ounces
- 4 cups broccoli florets
- ½ teaspoon salt, divided
- ½ teaspoon ground black pepper, divided
- ¼ cup prepared pesto
- 2 tablespoons olive oil

- 1 medium tomato, sliced
- 3 ounces mozzarella cheese, halved, sliced, low-fat

Directions

- Switch on the oven, then set it to 375 degrees F and let it preheat.
- Meanwhile, prepare the chicken breasts and for this, make crosswise cuts in it, not all the way through, and at every ½ inch.
- Season each chicken breast with ¼ teaspoon each of salt and black pepper and then stuff the cuts in chicken breasts alternately with a tomato slice and cheese slice.
- Take a large bowl, place broccoli florets in it, add remaining salt and black pepper, drizzle with oil and then toss until coated.
- Take a large baking sheet, place the prepared chicken breasts on one side of the baking sheet, and then scatter broccoli florets on the other side of the baking sheet.
- Bake the prepared chicken breasts and broccoli florets for 25 minutes or more until chicken has thoroughly cooked and broccoli turns tender, stirring broccoli halfway.
- When done, cut each chicken breast in half and then serve each chicken breast piece with one-fourth of the roasted broccoli florets.

Lentil, Chickpea and Tomato Soup

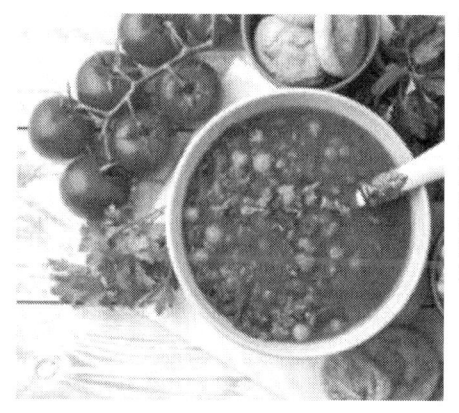

Nutritional Information per Serving

Calories: 291 calories
Fat: 9g
Sat. Fat: 1.5g
Carbohydrates: 42g
Protein: 12g
Fiber: 13.5g

Prep Time: 10 minutes | Cook Time: 35 minutes | Servings: 4

Ingredients

- ½ cup green lentils, uncooked, rinsed
- ¼ cup white whole-wheat flour
- 1 large white onion, peeled, sliced
- 1 stick of celery, chopped
- 1 cup cooked chickpeas
- 1 cup cilantro leaves
- 4 tomatoes, peeled
- 1 cup parsley leaves
- 1 teaspoon salt
- ½ cup whole-wheat thin pasta, broken in quarters
- 1 teaspoon turmeric powder
- 1 teaspoon ground black pepper
- ½ teaspoon ginger powder
- ½ piece of vegetable bouillon cube, salted
- 2 tablespoons olive oil
- 4 tablespoons tomato paste
- 6 ¼ cups water

Directions

- Plug in a food processor, add onion, celery, tomatoes, and ½ cup each of parsley and cilantro, and then pulse until smooth.
- Pour the mixture into a large pot, add 2 cups of water, place the pot over high heat and then bring it to a boil.
- Add ginger, lentils, bouillon cube, tomato paste, and olive oil, stir in salt, black pepper, and turmeric and then bring the soup to boil.
- Then switch heat to the low level, simmer the soup for 10 minutes, add pasta and chickpeas, pour in 4 cups water, bring the soup to boil, and then simmer for 5 minutes.
- Meanwhile, place flour in a blender, pour in the remaining water, and then pulse until smooth.
- After 5 minutes, slowly pour the flour mixture into the pot, stirring continuously, and then simmer for another 5 minutes.
- When done, add remaining cilantro and parsley leaves, taste to adjust seasoning, and then remove the pot from heat.
- Ladle the soup among 4 bowls and then serve.

Greek Red Lentil Soup

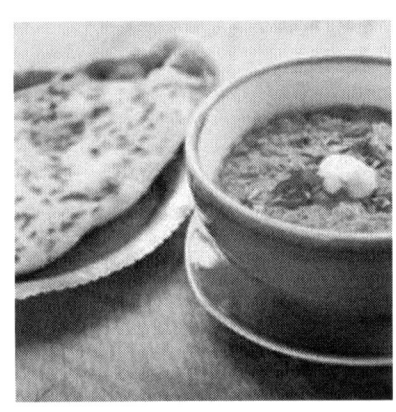

Nutritional Information per Serving

Calories: 293.3 calories
Fat: 4.5g
Sat. Fat: 1.2g
Carbohydrates: 47.4g
Protein: 15.8g
Fiber: 9.4g

Prep Time: 10 minutes | Cook Time: 30 minutes | Servings: 4; 1 bowl per serving

Ingredients

- 1 medium white onion, peeled, chopped
- ¾ cup crushed tomatoes
- 1 medium carrot, peeled, chopped
- 1 tablespoon minced garlic
- 2 teaspoons dried oregano
- 1 ½ cups red lentils, uncooked, rinsed, drained
- 1 teaspoon ground cumin
- ½ teaspoon dried rosemary
- 1 teaspoon salt
- ½ teaspoon red pepper flakes
- 2 bay leaves
- ½ of a lemon, zested
- 2 tablespoons olive oil
- 1 lemon, juiced
- 4 cups vegetable broth
- 4 tablespoons parsley leaves
- 4 tablespoons crumbled feta cheese, low-fat

Directions

- Take a large pot, place it over medium-high heat, add oil, and when hot, add onion, garlic, and carrots, and then cook for 4 minutes until vegetables begin to soften.
- Add oregano, cumin, oregano, rosemary, red pepper flakes, and bay leaves, and then cook for 1 minute until fragrant.
- Add lentils and tomatoes, pour in the broth, stir in salt and then bring the soup to a boil.
- Then switch heat to medium level and simmer the soup for 15 to 20 minutes until thoroughly cooked, covering the pot with its lid.
- When lentils have cooked, remove the pot from heat and then pulse it using an immersion blender until smooth and creamy.
- Return the pot over medium heat, cook for 3 to 4 minutes until thoroughly hot, and then stir in parsley, lemon zest, and juice.
- Divide the soup evenly among four bowls, drizzle with oil, top with feta cheese and then serve.

Greek Pasta

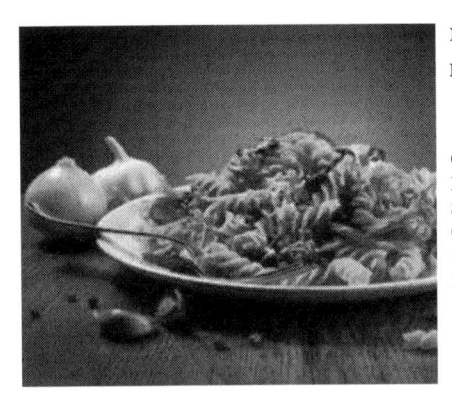

Nutritional Information per Serving

Calories: 308.3 calories
Fat: 8.7g
Sat. Fat: 3.1g
Carbohydrates: 40.4g
Protein: 17.1g
Fiber: 6g

Prep Time: 10 minutes | Cook Time: 25 minutes | Servings: 4

Ingredients

- 2 cups whole-wheat pasta
- 2 links of cooked chicken sausage, sliced into rounds
- ¾ cup diced white onion
- ½ teaspoon minced garlic
- 3 cups baby spinach
- 3 tablespoons chopped pitted Kalamata olives
- 1 ½ tablespoon olive oil
- 4 tablespoons crumbled feta cheese, low-fat
- 6 ounces canned tomato sauce, no-salt-added
- 3 tablespoons chopped basil

Directions

- Prepare the pasta, and for this, take a large pot half full with water, place it over medium-high heat and then bring it to a boil.

- Add the pasta, cook it for 8 to 10 minutes until tender, then drain it well and reserve ½ cup of a cooking liquid, set aside until required.
- Then take a large skillet pan, place it over medium-high heat, add oil, and when hot, add onion, sausage slices, and garlic, stir until mixed, and then cook for 4 to 6 minutes until onion begins to brown.
- Add the cooked pasta along with spinach, olives, and tomato sauce, stir until just mixed, and then cook for 3 to 5 minutes until spinach wilts and the sauce begins to bubble.
- Stir in basil leaves and feta cheese, then divide the prepared pasta evenly among four plates and serve.

Italian Minestrone Soup

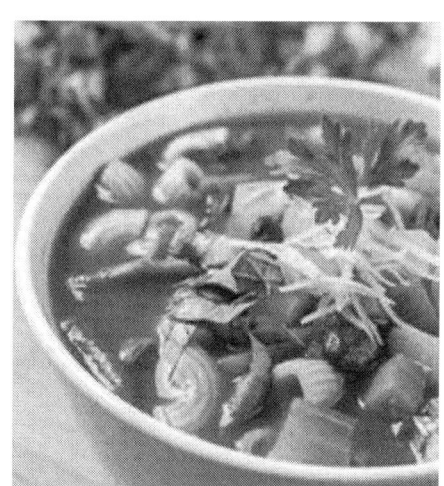

Nutritional Information per Serving

Calories: 301.7 calories
Fat: 9.3g
Sat. Fat: 2.5g
Carbohydrates: 39.7g
Protein: 14.8g
Fiber: 9.4g

Prep Time: 10 minutes | Cook Time: 40 minutes | Servings: 4; 1 bowl per serving

Ingredients

- 2 cups cooked small whole-wheat pasta
- 1 cup green beans, ends trimmed, cut into 1-inch pieces
- 1 small white onion, peeled, chopped
- 2 tablespoons minced garlic
- 15 ounces cooked kidney beans
- 2 medium carrots, peeled, chopped
- 1 large zucchini, ends trimmed, diced
- 2 celery stalks, diced
- 15 ounces crushed tomatoes

- 1 teaspoon salt
- ½ teaspoon ground black pepper
- 1 teaspoon paprika
- 2 sprigs of thyme
- ½ teaspoon dried rosemary
- ¼ cup chopped parsley
- 1 bay leaf
- ¼ cup olive oil
- ¼ cup basil leaves
- 6 cups vegetable broth
- 4 tablespoons grated Parmesan cheese, low-fat

Directions

- Take a large pot, place it over medium-high heat, add oil, and when hot, add onion, celery, and carrots, and then cook for 5 minutes until vegetables begin to soften.
- Stir in garlic, cook for 1 minute, add green beans and zucchini, and then stir in rosemary, paprika, and ¼ teaspoon each of salt and black pepper until combined.
- Add tomatoes, bay leaf, and thyme, pour in the broth, bring it to a boil, then switch heat to medium-low level and simmer the soup for 20 minutes, covering the pot with its lid.
- Add kidney beans, continue cooking for 10 minutes and then stir in basil and parsley.
- Then add the cooked pasta, simmer for 2 to 3 minutes until thoroughly hot, and then remove the bay leaf.
- Taste the soup to adjust seasoning, remove the pot from heat, divide the soup evenly among four bowls and then serve.

Roasted Tomato and Basil Soup

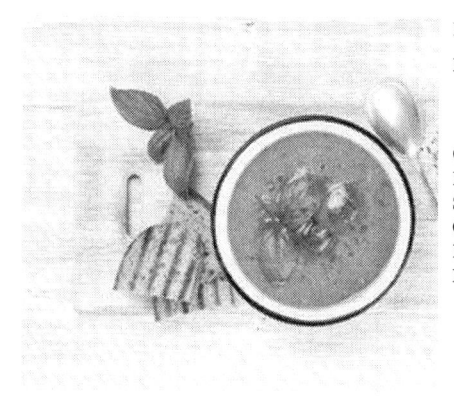

Nutritional Information per Serving

Calories: 322 calories
Fat: 16.8g
Sat. Fat: 3.1g
Carbohydrates: 33.4g
Protein: 9.3g
Fiber: 6.4g

Prep Time: 20 minutes | Cook Time: 1 hour | Servings: 4; 1 bowl per serving

Ingredients

- 2 pounds tomatoes, halved
- 2 medium white onions, chopped
- 1 teaspoon salt
- 4 cloves of garlic, peeled, minced
- 2/3 teaspoon dried thyme
- 2 medium carrots, peeled, diced
- 2/3 teaspoon dried oregano
- 2/3 cup crushed tomatoes
- 3/4 teaspoon ground black pepper
- 1/3 teaspoon ground cumin
- 1-ounce fresh basil leaves
- 1/3 teaspoon paprika
- 4 tablespoons olive oil
- 1 3/4 cup water

For Serving:
- 8 slices of whole-wheat French baguette, each about 1-inch thick
- 1 1/2 teaspoon minced garlic
- 1 1/2 teaspoon Italian herb seasoning
- 3/4 cup butter, unsalted, melted
- 1/4 teaspoon ground red pepper

Directions

- Switch on the oven, then set it to 450 degrees F and let it preheat.
- Meanwhile, take a large bowl, place carrot pieces and tomato halves in it, drizzle with 2 tablespoons of oil, season with ¼ teaspoon each of salt and black pepper, and then toss until combined.
- Take a large baking sheet, spread the vegetable mixture in a single layer, and then roast for 30 minutes until tender, stirring halfway.
- When done, let the vegetables cool for 10 minutes, transfer them to a blender, add ¼ cup water and then pulse until blended.
- Take a large pot, place it over medium-high heat, add remaining oil and when hot, add onions and then cook for 3 minutes or until beginning to tender.
- Add garlic, cook for 1 minute until fragrant, add the blended tomato-carrot mixture, crushed tomatoes, basil, cumin, paprika, thyme, and remaining salt, black pepper, and water, and then stir until mixed.
- Bring the soup to boil, then switch heat to low level and simmer for 20 to 30 minutes until soup has reached to desired consistency, covering the pot partway with its lid.
- While the soup cooks, grill the bread slices, and for this, place the butter in a medium heatproof bowl and then microwave for 1 to 2 minutes until melted, stirring every 30 seconds.
- Add Italian herb seasoning, garlic, and red pepper into the melted butter and then stir until combined.
- Take a griddle pan, place it over medium-high heat and let it preheat.
- Working on one baguette slice at a time, dip both sides in the prepared butter mixture or brush the butter mixture generously on both pieces of bread and then place it on the griddle pan.
- Add more buttered bread slices in the griddle pan until filled and then grill for 2 to 3 minutes per side until nicely golden brown and developed grill marks.
- When done, divide the tomato soup evenly among four bowls, drizzle some more olive oil on top and then serve each bowl with 2 toasted slices of whole-wheat French baguette.

Chapter 10

Desserts

Olive Oil Gelato

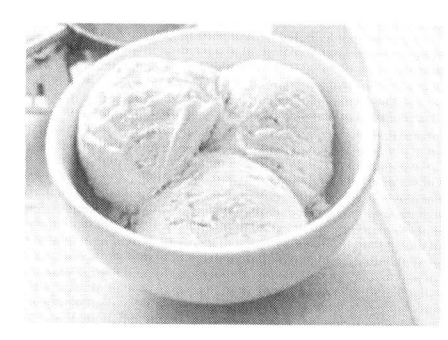

Nutritional Information per Serving

Calories: 234 calories
Fat: 18.4g
Sat. Fat: 4.2g
Carbohydrates: 14g
Protein: 2.9g
Fiber: 0.3g

Prep Time: 7 hours | Cook Time: 15 minutes | Servings: 4; 1 bowl per serving

Ingredients

- ¾ cup coconut sugar
- 4 egg yolks, at room temperature
- 1/8 teaspoon salt
- ¼ cup and 2 tablespoons water
- ¼ cup olive oil
- ¾ cup coconut milk, unsweetened, low-fat

Directions

- Take a medium pot, pour in the water and milk, and then stir in salt and sugar until mixed.
- Place the pot over medium heat and then cook for 3 to 5 minutes until bubbles form around the edges of the pot.
- Meanwhile, take a large bowl, fill it with ice, place another bowl on the ice and set it aside until required.
- Take a separate large bowl, place egg yolks in it and then whisk until frothy.
- Then whisk in the milk mixture in a steady stream until combined, and then pour this mixture into the pot.
- Switch heat to a low level and cook the custard until it has thickened enough to coat the back of a spoon or its temperature reaches 185 degrees F, stirring continuously.
- Then immediately spoon the custard into the bowl placed over ice, and then stir the custard until cooled.
- When cooled, cover the custard bowl with its lid, place it into the refrigerator and let it chill overnight.
- Then whisk oil into the custard in a steady stream until smooth, cover the bowl with its lid, and place it in the refrigerator for 6 hours, stirring every 1 hour.
- You can also churn the custard in an ice cream maker.
- When ready to eat, let the gelato rest for 15 minutes at room temperature, scoop it into bowls, and then serve.

Chocolate Avocado Mousse

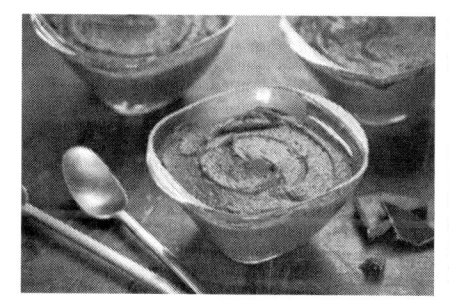

Nutritional Information per Serving

Calories: 240 calories
Fat: 12.7g
Sat. Fat: 2g
Carbohydrates: 28.1g
Protein: 2.9g
Fiber: 9.8g

Prep Time: 35 minutes | Cook Time: 0 minutes | Servings: 4; 1 bowl per serving

Ingredients

- 2 avocados, peeled, pitted
- 6 tablespoons date syrup
- 1 banana, peeled
- ½ teaspoon vanilla extract, unsweetened
- ¼ cup cocoa powder, unsweetened
- 1 tablespoon almond butter, unsalted
- 2 tablespoons almond milk, low-fat, unsweetened
- Berries as needed for topping

Directions

- Peel the bananas, cut them into pieces, and add them to a blender.
- Cut avocado into slices, add to the blender along with almond butter, date syrup, vanilla, and milk, and then pulse until combined.
- Divide the mousse evenly among four bowls, place them in the refrigerator and let them chill for 30 minutes or until required.

- When ready to eat, top the mousse with berries or favorite fruits and then serve.

Rice Pudding with Almond Milk

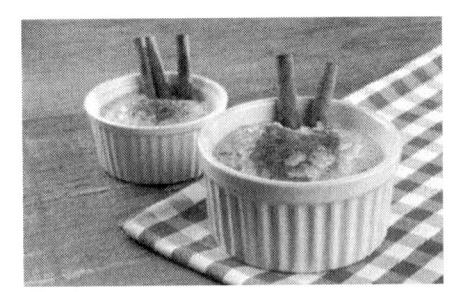

Nutritional Information per Serving

Calories: 257 calories
Fat: 6.3g
Sat. Fat: 0.7g
Carbohydrates: 41.7g
Protein: 8.3g
Fiber: 3.6g

Prep Time: 10 minutes | Cook Time: 30 minutes | Servings: 4; 1 bowl per serving

Ingredients

- 1/3 cup Medjool dates, pitted
- 1/3 cup whole raisins
- ¾ cup brown rice, uncooked
- ½ teaspoon vanilla extract, unsweetened
- ¼ toasted and chopped, sliced almonds
- ¼ teaspoon almond extract, unsweetened
- 1/8 teaspoon ground cinnamon
- 3 cups almond milk, vanilla flavor, unsweetened, low-fat
- 1/3 cup boiling water

Directions

- Prepare the date syrup and for this, take a medium bowl, place dates in it, pour in the boiling water, and let them soak for 15 minutes.

- Then transfer the dates with water into a food processor and pulse until smooth, set aside until required.
- Take a medium saucepan, place rice in it, pour in the milk, and then bring the mixture to a boil.
- Switch heat to medium-low level, simmer the rice for 20 to 30 minutes until rice has absorbed all the milk, stirring occasionally.
- Then add almonds, raisins, cinnamon, prepared date syrup, and vanilla, and almond extract and stir until mixed.
- Divide the pudding evenly among four bowls and then serve.

Vanilla Baked Pears

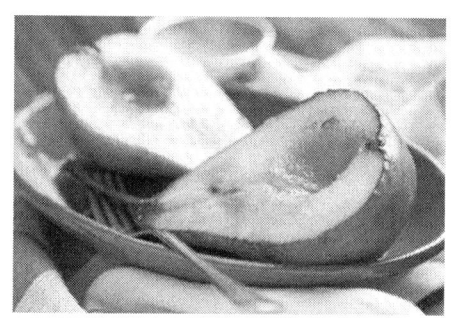

Nutritional Information per Serving

Calories: 216 calories
Fat: 0.5g
Sat. Fat: 0.25g
Carbohydrates: 50.6g
Protein: 2.1g
Fiber: 6.6g

Prep Time: 10 minutes | Cook Time: 25 minutes | Servings: 4; 2 pear halves per serving

Ingredients

- 4 medium pears
- ½ cup date syrup
- ¼ teaspoon ground cinnamon
- 1 teaspoon vanilla extract, unsweetened
- 4 tablespoons Greek yogurt, low-fat

Directions

- Switch on the oven, then set it to 375 degrees F and let it preheat.
- Meanwhile, cut each pear in half, remove its core using a small cookie scoop, and then cut a little piece from the bottom to make pear halves stand upright on a baking sheet.
- Take a large baking sheet, arrange pear halves in it cut-side-up and then sprinkle with cinnamon.
- Take a small bowl, place vanilla extract and date syrup in it, whisk until combined, and then drizzle over the prepared pear halves, reserving 2 tablespoons of the syrup for later use.
- Place the prepared baking sheet into the oven and bake the pears for 25 minutes until the edges turn golden brown.
- When done, drizzle the reserved maple syrup over the roasted pears and then divide pear halves among four plates, 2 pear halves per plate.
- Add 1 tablespoon yogurt to each plate and then serve.

Strawberry Popsicles

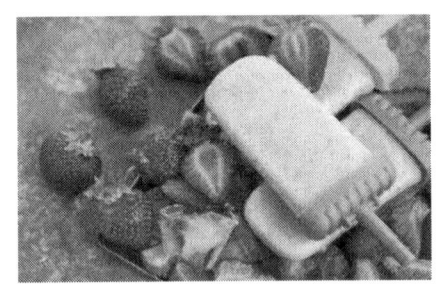

Nutritional Information per Serving

Calories: 38 calories
Fat: 0.6g
Sat. Fat: 0.05g
Carbohydrates: 6.9g
Protein: 0.6g
Fiber: 1.9g

Prep Time: 4 hours and 10 minutes | Cook Time: 0 minutes | Servings: 4; 1 popsicle per serving

Ingredients

- 2 ½ cups strawberries, fresh, rinsed
- ½ cup almond milk, unsweetened, low-fat

Directions

- Wash the berries and using a small sharp knife, remove the hull from each berry and discard it.
- Place the strawberries into a blender, pour in the milk, and then pulse until smooth.
- Divide the berries mixture evenly among the four popsicle molds, place a stick into each popsicle and then place the popsicle molds in a freezer.
- Let the popsicle freeze for a minimum of 4 hours or until firm and then serve.

Coconut, Tahini, and Cashew Bars

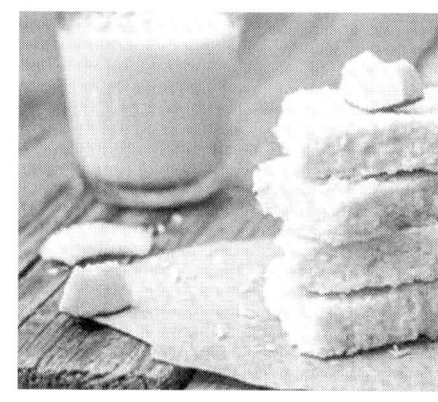

Nutritional Information per Serving

Calories: 155 calories
Fat: 11.8g
Sat. Fat: 4.3g
Carbohydrates: 8.7g
Protein: 2.6g
Fiber: 1.6g

Prep Time: 35 minutes | Cook Time: 0 minutes | Servings: 8; 2 bars per serving

Ingredients

For the Base:
- 2 Medjool dates, pitted
- ⅛ teaspoon salt
- ¼ cup walnuts
- ½ tablespoon coconut oil
- 2 tablespoons cashews

For the Filling:
- ¼ cup dried coconut, unsweetened, more as needed for sprinkling
- ¼ cup cashew butter
- ¼ teaspoon ground cinnamon
- 2 tablespoons tahini (prepared from the 'Sauces, Dips, and Dressing' section)
- ⅛ teaspoon salt
- ½ tablespoon coconut oil

Directions

- Take a small bowl, place the pitted dates in it, cover with warm water, and then let the dates rest for 5 minutes or more until softened.
- Then drain the dates, add them into the blender, add salt, nuts, oil, and cashews and then pulse until combined and the mixture resembles dough.
- Take a square bread pan, line it with a parchment sheet, spoon the date mixture in it, spread it evenly, then place the pan into a freezer and then let it rest for 10 minutes.
- Meanwhile, prepare the filling and for this, place all of its ingredients in a blender and then pulse until smooth.
- Spoon the prepared filling mixture into the prepared bread pan, spread it evenly, and then sprinkle some more coconut on top.
- Return the bread pan into the freezer and let it freeze for another 15 minutes.
- Then take out the crust by pulling it out using the parchment sheet and then cut the crust into 1-inch rectangle-sized bars.
- Transfer the bars into an air-tight container and store them in a freezer until ready to eat.

Applesauce Oat Muffins

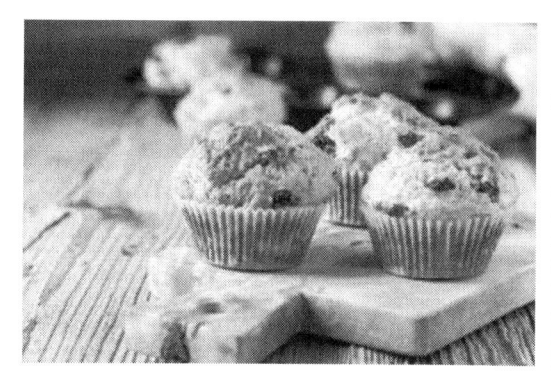

Nutritional Information per Serving

Calories: 196 calories
Fat: 1.1g
Sat. Fat: 0.3g
Carbohydrates: 24.6g
Protein: 23.5g
Fiber: 1.8g

Prep Time: 10 minutes | Cook Time: 20 minutes | Servings: 4 muffins; 1 muffin per serving

Ingredients

- ½ cup old-fashioned rolled oats
- 6 tablespoons whole-wheat flour
- ½ teaspoon baking powder
- ½ teaspoon ground cinnamon
- 3 tablespoons coconut sugar
- 1/3 teaspoon baking soda
- 1/8 teaspoon salt
- ½ cup applesauce, unsweetened
- 1 ½ tablespoon melted coconut oil
- 3 tablespoons almond milk, unsweetened, low-fat
- ½ teaspoon vanilla extract, unsweetened
- ¼ cup raisins
- ½ of a large egg

Directions

- Switch on the oven, then set it to 375 degrees F and let it preheat.
- Take 4 large silicone muffin cups, grease them with oil, and set aside until required.
- Take a medium bowl, place oats, sugar, egg, and coconut oil, pour in milk and applesauce and stir until well combined.
- Take another medium bowl, place whole-wheat flour in it, add salt, baking powder, cinnamon, baking soda, and raisins and then stir until mixed.
- Slowly stir in oats mixture until incorporated and then divide the batter evenly among four prepared silicone muffin cups.
- Place the prepared muffin cups in the oven and then bake for 15 to 20 minutes until firm and the top turns golden brown.
- When done, let the muffins cool in their cups for 10 minutes, then take them out and cool completely before serving.

Baked Apple Slices

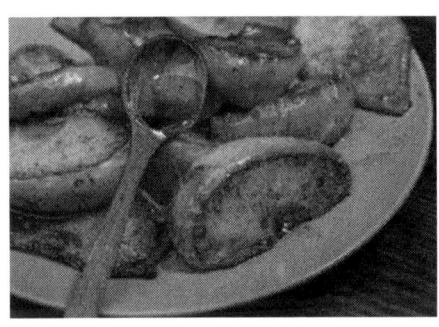

Nutritional Information per Serving

Calories: 228 calories
Fat: 10.5g
Sat. Fat: 8g
Carbohydrates: 32g
Protein: 1g
Fiber: 3g

Prep Time: 10 minutes | Cook Time: 20 minutes | Servings: 4

Ingredients

- 4 large apples, unpeeled
- 4 teaspoons ground cinnamon
- 4 tablespoons cashew butter, unsalted, melted

Directions

- Switch on the oven, then set it to 400 degrees F and let it preheat.
- Meanwhile, take a square rimmed baking sheet about 8-inches, line it with a parchment sheet, and set it aside until required.
- Cut each apple in half, remove its core, and then slice each apple half into six pieces, each about ¼-inch thick.
- Scatter the apple pieces in a single layer, drizzle with melted butter, toss them until coated, and then spread the apple pieces in a single layer.
- Sprinkle 2 teaspoons of cinnamon on top of apple slices and then bake the apples for 10 minutes.
- Then flip the apple pieces, sprinkle the remaining cinnamon on top, and then continue baking for 10 minutes until apple slices turn tender and nicely golden brown.
- Serve straight away.

Chocolate Dipped Strawberries

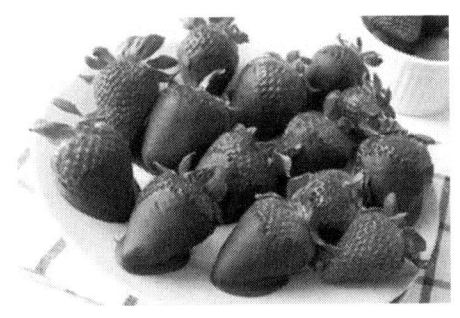

Nutritional Information per Serving

Calories: 235 calories
Fat: 16g
Sat. Fat: 6g
Carbohydrates: 18g
Protein: 4g
Fiber: 4g

Prep Time: 45 minutes | Cook Time: 2 minutes | Servings: 12 strawberries; 4 strawberries per serving

Ingredients

- 12 strawberries, fresh, rinsed
- 1 tablespoon cashew butter, unsalted
- 1 cup chocolate chips, unsweetened
- 1 teaspoon sesame seeds

Directions

- Take a medium heatproof bowl, place chocolate chips, and then microwave for 1 to 2 minutes until chocolate has melted, stirring every 30 seconds.
- Take a large baking sheet, line it with a parchment sheet, and set aside until required.
- Working on one strawberry at a time, hold it from its stem, and then dip it into the melted chocolate to coat it.
- Place the strawberry on the prepared baking sheet, sprinkle some sesame seeds on the coated strawberry and then repeat with the remaining berries.

- Place the prepared baking sheet containing berries in a refrigerator, let it rest for 40 minutes until chocolate has firmed, and then serve.

Watermelon and Mint Granita

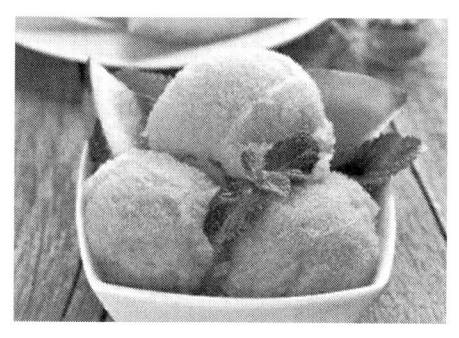

Nutritional Information per Serving

Calories: 168 calories
Fat: 0.4g
Sat. Fat: 0.04g
Carbohydrates: 39.2g
Protein: 1.2g
Fiber: 2.4g

Prep Time: 3 hours and 30 minutes | Cook Time: 0 minutes | Servings: 4; 1 bowl per serving

Ingredients

- 8 cups watermelon cubes, deseeded
- 3 limes, juiced
- 6 tablespoons coconut sugar
- 2 tablespoons mint leaves, chopped
- ½ teaspoon peppermint extract, unsweetened

Directions

- Place the watermelon pieces in a food processor and then pulse until smooth.
- Take a large bowl, place a fine sieve on it and then pass through the watermelon mixture and then discard the solids.
- Add lime juice into the collected watermelon mixture, add mint, sugar, and peppermint extract and then stir until sugar has dissolved.

- Take a 9-by-13 inches metal baking pan, pour the watermelon mixture in it, place it in the freezer and let it rest for 30 minutes.
- Remove the baking pan from the freezer, scrape granita using a fork, return it into the freezer for 3 hours, scrape granita every 30 minutes and then serve.

Peach Soup

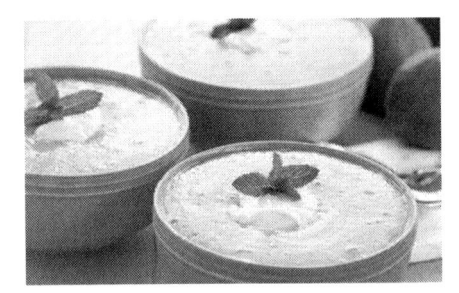

Nutritional Information per Serving

Calories: 258 calories
Fat: 17.2g
Sat. Fat: 4.3g
Carbohydrates: 21.3g
Protein: 4.5g
Fiber: 3.1g

Prep Time: 1 hour and 5 minutes | Cook Time: 0 minutes | Servings: 4

Ingredients

- 3 cups sliced peaches
- ¼ cup cucumber pieces, peeled
- ½ teaspoon salt
- 1 clove of garlic, peeled
- ¼ teaspoon ground black pepper
- ¼ cup green bell pepper pieces
- 2 tablespoons honey, raw
- ¼ cup balsamic vinegar
- 3 tablespoons goat cheese, low-fat, and more as needed for topping
- ¼ cup water
- ¼ cup olive oil and more as needed

Directions

- Place peaches, green bell pepper, and cucumber pieces in a blender, and then add garlic, salt, black pepper, honey, vinegar, and goat cheese.
- Pour in the water and oil, pulse until well combined, and then pour the soup into a large bowl.
- Taste it to adjust seasoning, then cover the soup bowl with its lid, place it in the refrigerator and let it rest for 1 hour until cold.
- When ready to eat, divide the soup evenly among four bowls, top with some goat cheese, drizzle with some oil and then serve.

Grilled Watermelon Salad

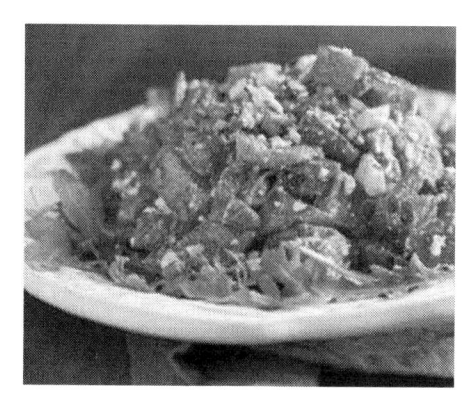

Nutritional Information per Serving

Calories: 171 calories
Fat: 7.05g
Sat. Fat: 2.4g
Carbohydrates: 20.4g
Protein: 5.4g
Fiber: 1.1g

Prep Time: 20 minutes | Cook Time: 8 minutes | Servings: 4; 1 bowl per serving

Ingredients

- 1 small watermelon
- 4 leaves of basil, chopped
- 4 leaves of mint
- 1 tablespoon olive oil

- 1 lemon, juiced, zested
- ½ cup grated parmesan cheese

Directions

- Prepare the watermelon and for this, cut it into quarters and then cut each piece into ½-inch thick triangles.
- Take a griddle pan, place it over medium-high heat and let it preheat until hot.
- Brush the watermelon triangle pieces with oil, arrange them on the griddle pan and then cook for 3 to 4 minutes per side or more until grill marks appear.
- When done, transfer the watermelon pieces to a plate, cool them for 10 minutes, peel the rind and then chop the watermelon flesh.
- Transfer the chopped watermelon to a medium bowl, add basil, mint, lemon juice and zest, and cheese, and then stir until combined.
- Divide the salad evenly among four bowls and then serve.

Leave a 1-click review!

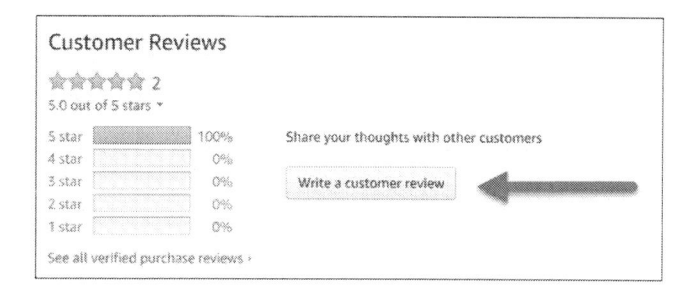

I would be incredibly grateful if you take just 60 seconds to write just a brief review on Amazon, even if it's just a few sentences.

https://www.amazon.com/review/create-review-asin=B09MJ5282Q

Conclusion

Our lives are short and fleeting and therefore, we have a responsibility to make it count. We owe it to us and to our bodies that work relentlessly to keep us alive and healthy. We should not return all the unhealthy compounds in response to the healthy equilibrium that our biological system tries to maintain every single second of the day. Take a seat and think how unjust we have been to our bodies. It will fill your eyes in tears because millions and trillions of cells work together to keep us alive and healthy. Is that how we are returning the favor? We are living in times where we are constantly taught to work longer and harder. Practicing a lifestyle like that gives us no time to think about what we eat to keep us going. We barely get enough time to stop and think about what needs to be changed in our eating patterns or what steps we need to take to adopt a new way of eating food. After juggling various diets, I finally understood that our food directly links with how efficiently we function in society, and I realized it when I switched to the Mediterranean diet. That's why this book, "Mediterranean Diet for Beginners," is a personal endeavor to make people realize that it is about time we eat healthily and give back to our bodies. By retreating to a healthy and prosperous living by transitioning to a Mediterranean diet, we can enjoy the perks of good health and tastes of nutritious food.

The Mediterranean diet is more than just what meets the eye. It is a way of living and loving to eat, and this diet is a prime instance of what a healthy diet regime should be. It allows the consumption of healthy and nutritious food coupled with sufficient exercise for a balanced life. The Mediterranean diet has been the favorite research area for nutrition scientists for decades, and every time, they end up discovering more benefits that further confirm that this diet should be the only standard healthy diet pattern for people to follow.

As mentioned previously, the discovery of the Mediterranean diet by Ancel Keys unlocked the door for the entire world to see how food impacts the quality of our lives. In addition, he unveiled the relationship between eating healthy and living longer. He also strived to make people understand the link between diet and severe health complications. Briefly speaking, the Mediterranean diet has been researched countless times on different population samples, healthy and ill alike. The results have further confirmed that it is the best regimen to ever exist. On a Mediterranean diet, health is defined in different ways. It does not limit health by being alive and able to work long hours without collapsing. Instead, it associates being healthy with aspects like what and how you eat, what kind of people you share meals with, how you utilize your free time, and lastly, how frequently you exercise? When your life lacks any of the listed components, you tend to suffer mentally, physically, and emotionally. All these factors combined, make up the basic principles of the Mediterranean diet.

And, being on a Mediterranean diet is like a stroke of warmth on a cold winter evening, and the warmth comes from eating with your loved ones, being in their heartwarming presence. The Mediterranean diet treats meal times as social events, where all the family members should gather at a dining table and enjoy their food together. So, do not treat the Mediterranean diet like a typical diet regimen. Instead, consider it like committing to the Mediterranean culture where eating healthy food is prized and valued, where meals are prepared with love and shared with people we care about.

As an author and a body fat expert with long experience of the Mediterranean diet, I have tried my very best to deliver information through this ebook about the Mediterranean way of life and potential benefits, backed by authentic scientific studies. In addition, we learned how to shop for the ingredients, so if you make up your mind to transition to the Mediterranean diet, you should know what ingredients to shop for and from where. You can start by making small changes because even the smallest ones make up a huge difference in the long term. Besides, now you know how to swap processed foods and replace them with healthy and more wholesome and nutritious foods. By now, you have learned that following the Mediterranean diet involves eating lots of fresh produce such as fruits, vegetables, specified types of meat, and little to moderate consumption of red wine. You have also learned what kind of fats you can consume or use for cooking; for instance, extra virgin olive oil is commonly used. Moreover, after reading this ebook, you have realized that following a Mediterranean diet is more about choosing to live healthy rather than solely losing weight. In addition, the section on meal portions and sizes is there to assist you in cooking calculated portions of meals so that no amount of food is wasted. Finally, by cooking the recipes shared in this ebook, you can invite friends over and share some of the best dinners filled with laughs, good people, and scrumptious foods.

If you find this book fun in exploring the diverse taste of the Mediterranean diet, please do share this experience by leaving your feedback on Amazon. Your review would be highly appreciated.

To your healthy living!

My other books you will love!

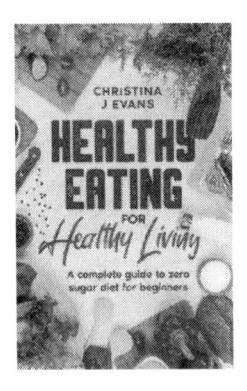

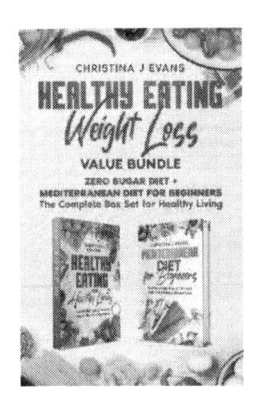

Amazon.com/dp/B09MCXR9T5

Amazon.com/dp/B09MHF2XQ1

Don't forget to grab your GIFT!!!

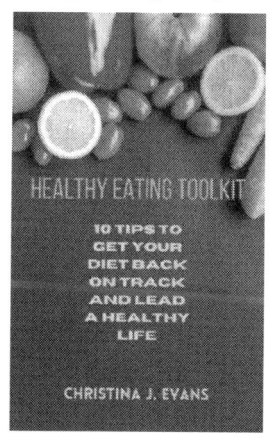

http://christinajevans.com/healthy-eating.pdf

Joining the HL Community

Looking to build your healthy eating lifestyle? If so, then check out the Healthy Living (HL) Community here:

www.facebook.com/groups/1004091000384321/

References

A. (2020a, February 20). *Mediterranean Diet Friendly Chocolate Dipped Strawberries*. Food Wine and Love. https://foodwineandlove.com/mediterranean-diet-friendly-chocolate-dipped-strawberries/

A. (2020b, March 20). *Oil Free Baked Veggie Chips (Paleo, Vegan, Gluten Free)*. The Big Man's World ®. https://thebigmansworld.com/oil-free-baked-veggie-chips-paleo-vegan-gluten-free/#recipe

A. (2020c, March 24). *Mediterranean Diet Ranch Dressing*. Food Wine and Love. https://foodwineandlove.com/mediterranean-diet-ranch-dressing/

A. (2020d, April 20). *Mediterranean Diet Shrimp in Garlic Sauce*. Food Wine and Love. https://foodwineandlove.com/mediterranean-diet-shrimp-in-garlic-sauce/

A. (2020e, October 5). *Chocolate Mousse (no dairy)*. The Mediterranean Movement. https://www.themedimove.com/recipes/diet-recipes/desserts/chocolate-avocado-mousse/

A. (2021a, August 23). *Homemade Trail Mix -*. Fully Mediterranean. https://fullymediterranean.com/recipes/homemade-trail-mix/

Allen, L. (2021, September 8). *Healthy Applesauce Oat Muffins*. Tastes Better From Scratch. https://tastesbetterfromscratch.com/healthy-applesauce-oat-muffins/#recipe

Almond and Brown Rice Pudding. (n.d.). Whole Foods Market. Retrieved October 12, 2021, from https://eu.wholefoodsmarket.com/?destination=www.wholefoodsmarket.com%2Frecipes%2Falmond-brown-rice-pudding

Baked Eggs in Avocado. (2019, April 3). Allrecipes. https://www.allrecipes.com/recipe/240744/paleo-baked-eggs-in-avocado/

Barydakis, K. (2021, September 15). *Tzatziki Sauce: Greek Yogurt, Cucumber, Dill and Garlic*. Mediterranean Living. https://www.mediterraneanliving.com/tzatziki/

Berkowitz, S. F. (2016a, April 29). *Amba pickled mango sauce*. From the Grapevine. https://www.fromthegrapevine.com/israeli-kitchen/recipes/amba-pickled-mango-sauce

Berkowitz, S. F. (2016b, May 2). *Matbucha*. From the Grapevine. https://www.fromthegrapevine.com/israeli-kitchen/recipes/matbucha

Blackberry-Ginger Overnight Bulgur. (2016, August 17). Better Homes & Gardens. https://www.bhg.com/recipe/blackberry-ginger-overnight-bulgur/

Blueberry Lemon Breakfast Quinoa. (2012, December 20). Allrecipes. https://www.allrecipes.com/recipe/230830/blueberry-lemon-breakfast-quinoa/

Bradley, R. B. D. (2021a, September 15). *Balsamic Dill Yogurt Dressing*. Mediterranean Living. https://www.mediterraneanliving.com/balsamic-dill-yogurt-dressing/

Bradley, R. B. D. (2021b, September 15). *Bean Burgers with Garlic and Sage (Vegetarian, Gluten-Free)*. Mediterranean Living. https://www.mediterraneanliving.com/bean-burgers-garlic-sage-vegetarian-gluten-free/

Bradley, R. B. D. (2021c, September 15). *Tangy Italian Salad Dressing*. Mediterranean Living. https://www.mediterraneanliving.com/tangy-italian-salad-dressing/

Bradley, R. B. D. (2021d, October 11). *Mediterranean Fish Stew (30 minute recipe)*. Mediterranean Living. https://www.mediterraneanliving.com/mediterranean-fish-stew-30-minute-recipe/

Bradley, R. B. D. (2021e, October 12). *Cherry Tomato Sauce made in a Mason Jar*. Mediterranean Living. https://www.mediterraneanliving.com/cherry-tomato-sauce-made-in-a-mason-jar/

Cherry-Walnut Overnight Oats. (2018, December 14). EatingWell. https://www.eatingwell.com/recipe/269656/cherry-walnut-overnight-oats/

D. (2020f, January 29). *Italian Salsa Verde Recipe*. Our Salty Kitchen. https://oursaltykitchen.com/italian-salsa-verde/

Delgado, A. M., Almeida, M. D. V., & Parisi, S. (2017). *Chemistry of the Mediterranean diet*. Switzerland: Springer.

DeLeeuw, V. (2021, August 13). *Baked Apple Slices*. Healthy Recipes Blog. https://healthyrecipesblogs.com/baked-apple-slices-recipe/

Devinat, M. (2021a, September 23). *Spinach and Goat Cheese Quiche (France)*. Mediterranean Living. https://www.mediterraneanliving.com/spinach-and-goat-cheese-quiche-france/

Devinat, M. (2021b, September 23). *Tuna Patties Fried in Olive Oil (France)*. Mediterranean Living. https://www.mediterraneanliving.com/tuna-patties-fried-in-olive-oil-france/

Estruch, R., & Ros, E. (2020). *The role of the Mediterranean diet on weight loss and obesity-related diseases*. Reviews in Endocrine and Metabolic Disorders, 21(3), 315-327.

Ezzammoury, M. (2021, September 23). *Moroccan Harira (Lentil, Chickpea and Tomato Soup)*. Mediterranean Living. https://www.mediterraneanliving.com/moroccan-harira-lentil-chickpea-and-tomato-soup/

Feel Good Foodie. (2021, June 5). *Avocado Toast with Egg - 4 Ways*. FeelGoodFoodie. https://feelgoodfoodie.net/recipe/avocado-toast-with-egg-3-ways/#wprm-recipe-container-8175

Fontana, G. (2021a, September 23). *Italian Red Pesto with Sun-Dried Tomatoes and Arugula*. Mediterranean Living. https://www.mediterraneanliving.com/italian-red-pesto-with-sun-dried-tomatoes-and-arugula/

Fontana, G. (2021b, September 23). *Pesto Genovese (Traditional Italian Pesto)*. Mediterranean Living. https://www.mediterraneanliving.com/pesto-genovese-traditional-italian-pesto/

Fontana, G. (2021c, September 23). *Vegetarian Pasta Carbonara*. Mediterranean Living. https://www.mediterraneanliving.com/vegetable-carbonara/

Gib, J. (2006, September 13). *Mediterranean Fruit Salad Recipe - Food.com*. Food. https://www.food.com/recipe/mediterranean-fruit-salad-186006

Greek Turkey Burgers with Spinach, Feta & Tzatziki. (2018, February 6). EatingWell. https://www.eatingwell.com/recipe/262569/greek-turkey-burgers-with-spinach-feta-tzatziki/

Greek-Style Frittata. (2014, September 1). Better Homes & Gardens. https://www.bhg.com/recipe/greek-style-frittata/

H. (2021b, May 23). *Mediterranean Black Bean Salad With Herbs & Feta.* Homemade Mastery. https://www.homemademastery.com/mediterranean-black-bean-salad-with-herbs-feta/

HasanzadeNemati, S. (2021, May 3). *Mediterranean Baked Dijon Salmon Recipe [Video].* Unicorns in the Kitchen. https://www.unicornsinthekitchen.com/mediterranean-baked-dijon-salmon-recipe-video/#recipe/

Hasselback Caprese Chicken. (2017, November 16). EatingWell. https://www.eatingwell.com/recipe/261639/hasselback-caprese-chicken/

Hesser, A. (2019, August 20). *Olive Oil Gelato.* Food52. https://food52.com/recipes/10866-olive-oil-gelato

K. (2019a, January 31). *Mediterranean Roasted Chickpeas Recipe.* A Simple Pantry. https://asimplepantry.com/roasted-chickpeas-recipe/

K. (2020g, May 22). *Best Tahini Sauce.* Cookie and Kate. https://cookieandkate.com/best-tahini-sauce-recipe/

Kale Chips. (n.d.). Carb Manager. Retrieved October 12, 2021, from https://www.carbmanager.com/recipe-detail/ug:9977456c-74f2-45e2-24e2-3959d917652b/keto-mediterranean-kale-chips

L. (2021c, April 2). *Easy Homemade Flatbread Crackers.* Pinch of Yum. https://pinchofyum.com/easy-homemade-flatbread-crackers

LeBlanc, G. (2021, September 15). *Baked Cod with Sun-Dried Tomatoes and Olives.* Mediterranean Living. https://www.mediterraneanliving.com/baked-cod-sun-dried-tomatoes-olives/

M. (2017, June 28). *Strawberry popsicles*. Tasty Mediterraneo. https://www.tastymediterraneo.com/strawberry-popsicles/

M. (2020h, March 2). *Mediterranean style guacamole*. Tasty Mediterraneo. https://www.tastymediterraneo.com/mediterranean-style-guacamole/

Martínez-González, M. Á., De la Fuente-Arrillaga, C., Nunez-Cordoba, J. M., Basterra-Gortari, F. J., Beunza, J. J., Vazquez, Z., ... & Bes-Rastrollo, M. (2008). *Adherence to Mediterranean diet and risk of developing diabetes: prospective cohort study*. Bmj, 336(7657), 1348-1351.

Martínez-González, M. Á., Hershey, M. S., Zazpe, I., & Trichopoulou, A. (2017). *Transferability of the Mediterranean diet to non-Mediterranean countries. What is and what is not the Mediterranean diet*. Nutrients, 9(11), 1226.

McDowell, B. (2021, March 3). *Chia Pomegranate Smoothie*. The Domestic Dietitian. https://thedomesticdietitian.com/chia-pomegranate-smoothie/

Mediterranean Cauliflower Pizza. (2016, June 3). EatingWell. https://www.eatingwell.com/recipe/250891/mediterranean-cauliflower-pizza/

Mediterranean Chickpea Quinoa Bowl. (2017, May 11). EatingWell. https://www.eatingwell.com/recipe/258195/mediterranean-chickpea-quinoa-bowl/

Mediterranean Grilled Sea Bass. (2021, April 30). Good Housekeeping. https://www.goodhousekeeping.com/food-recipes/a6026/mediterranean-grilled-sea-bass-2200/

Mediterranean Sweet and Sour Chicken. (2019, June 5). Good Housekeeping. https://www.goodhousekeeping.com/food-recipes/a5393/mediterranean-sweet-sour-chicken-1815/

Mindbody green. (2018, January 10). *Coconut, Tahini, and Cashew Bars*. https://www.mindbodygreen.com/articles/blood-sugar-balancing-tahini-dessert

Morris, N. A. D. (2021, September 15). *Yogurt Tahini Dip and Dressing*. Mediterranean Living. https://www.mediterraneanliving.com/yogurt-tahini-dip-and-dressing/

Murray, T., & Murray, T. (2021, June 7). *Shakshuka*. Good Housekeeping. https://www.goodhousekeeping.com/food-recipes/a34908201/easy-shakshuka-recipe/

One-Pot Greek Pasta. (2018, February 28). EatingWell. https://www.eatingwell.com/recipe/262954/one-pot-greek-pasta/

P. (2021d, August 23). *Peach Soup -*. Fully Mediterranean. https://fullymediterranean.com/recipes/peach-soup/

Paoli, A., Bianco, A., Grimaldi, K. A., Lodi, A., & Bosco, G. (2013). *Long term successful weight loss with a combination biphasic ketogenic mediterranean diet and mediterranean diet maintenance protocol.* Nutrients, 5(12), 5205-5217.

Pineapple Green Smoothie. (2016, June 3). EatingWell. https://www.eatingwell.com/recipe/251038/pineapple-green-smoothie/

Quinoa & Chia Oatmeal Mix. (2016, October 12). EatingWell. https://www.eatingwell.com/recipe/255762/quinoa-chia-oatmeal-mix/

Quinoa Avocado Salad. (2018, April 19). EatingWell. https://www.eatingwell.com/recipe/264061/quinoa-avocado-salad/

Rinaldi de Alvarenga, J. F., Quifer-Rada, P., Westrin, V., Hurtado-Barroso, S., Torrado-Prat, X., & Lamuela-Raventós, R. M. (2019*). Mediterranean sofrito home-cooking technique enhances polyphenol content in tomato sauce.* Journal of the Science of Food and Agriculture, 99(14), 6535-6545.

S. (2019b, December 30). *Tabouli Salad Recipe (Tabbouleh).* The Mediterranean Dish. https://www.themediterraneandish.com/tabouli-salad/

S. (2020i, April 17). *Crispy Homemade Fish Sticks.* The Mediterranean Dish. https://www.themediterraneandish.com/homemade-fish-sticks/

S. (2020j, May 17). *Easy Baba Ganoush Recipe.* The Mediterranean Dish. https://www.themediterraneandish.com/baba-ganoush-recipe/

S. (2020k, June 10). *Healthy Tomato, Basil, and Chickpea Salad - Vegan and Gluten-Free*. Beauty Bites. https://www.beautybites.org/healthy-tomatoes-basil-chickpea-salad-vegan-gluten-free/

S. (2020l, August 17). *Easy Roasted Tomato Basil Soup (Vegan, GF)*. The Mediterranean Dish. https://www.themediterraneandish.com/vegan-roasted-tomato-basil-soup/

S. (2020m, December 7). *Easy Greek Red Lentil Soup*. The Mediterranean Dish. https://www.themediterraneandish.com/red-lentil-soup-recipe/

S. (2020n, December 16). *Maple Vanilla Baked Pears*. Sally's Baking Addiction. https://sallysbakingaddiction.com/simple-maple-vanilla-baked-pears/

S. (2021e, January 6). *Creamy Tahini Date Banana Shake*. The Mediterranean Dish. https://www.themediterraneandish.com/tahini-date-banana-shake/

S. (2021f, February 1). *Baked Zucchini with Parmesan and Thyme*. The Mediterranean Dish. https://www.themediterraneandish.com/easy-baked-zucchini/

S. (2021g, March 20). *Simple Italian Minestrone Soup*. The Mediterranean Dish. https://www.themediterraneandish.com/simple-italian-minestrone-soup/

S. (2021h, September 3). *Mediterranean Grilled Chicken Kabobs*. The Mediterranean Dish. https://www.themediterraneandish.com/mediterranean-grilled-chicken-kabobs-tahini-sauce/

Sahyoun, N. R., & Sankavaram, K. (2016). *Historical origins of the Mediterranean diet, regional dietary profiles, and the development of the dietary guidelines*. In Mediterranean Diet (pp. 43-56). Humana Press, Cham.

Segrave-Daly, D. (2020, June 19). *Grilled Watermelon Salad: Grilled Fruit Recipe Roundup*. Teaspoon of Spice | Serena Ball MS, RD, & Deanna Segrave-Daly, RD. https://teaspoonofspice.com/grilled-watermelon-salad-grilled-fruit-recipes/

Stuffed Eggplant. (2016, June 3). EatingWell. https://www.eatingwell.com/recipe/253027/stuffed-eggplant/

Taste of Home Editors. (2021, September 25). *Mediterranean Shrimp Linguine*. Taste of Home. https://www.tasteofhome.com/recipes/mediterranean-shrimp-linguine/

Tercero, S. (2021, September 28). *Muhammara (Roasted Red Pepper and Walnut Dip)*. Mediterranean Living. https://www.mediterraneanliving.com/muhammara-roasted-red-pepper-and-walnut-dip/

Trichopoulou, A., & Vasilopoulou, E. (2000). *Mediterranean diet and longevity*. British Journal of Nutrition, 84(S2), S205-S209.

Watermelon and Mint Granita. (2017, August 10). The Best of Bridge. https://www.bestofbridge.com/watermelon-and-mint-granita/

Willett, W. C., Sacks, F., Trichopoulou, A., Drescher, G., Ferro-Luzzi, A., Helsing, E., & Trichopoulos, D. (1995). *Mediterranean diet pyramid: a cultural model for healthy eating*. The American journal of clinical nutrition, 61(6), 1402S-1406S.

Urquiaga, I., Echeverria, G., Dussaillant, C., & Rigotti, A. (2017). *Origin, components, and mechanisms of action of the Mediterranean diet*. Revista medica de Chile, 145(1), 85-95.

Yogurt with Blueberries & Honey. (2017, November 16). EatingWell. https://www.eatingwell.com/recipe/261617/yogurt-with-blueberries-honey/

Zikos, B. B. G. (2021, September 15). *Lebanese Hummus*. Mediterranean Living. https://www.mediterraneanliving.com/lebanese-hummus/

Zikos, G. (2021a, September 15). *Sheet Pan Baked Eggplant Parmesan*. Mediterranean Living. https://www.mediterraneanliving.com/sheet-pan-baked-eggplant-parmesan/

Zikos, G. (2021b, October 8). *Sheet Pan Chicken Thighs with Peppers and Onions*. Mediterranean Living. https://www.mediterraneanliving.com/sheet-pan-chicken-thighs-with-peppers-and-onions/

Zucchini with Egg. (2020, June 19). Allrecipes. https://www.allrecipes.com/recipe/242245/zucchini-with-egg/

Dump and Bake Chicken Fajita Bake With Quinoa - The ....
https://www.theseasonedmom.com/dump-bake-chicken-fajita-quinoa/

Printed in Great Britain
by Amazon